The Whiz Kid's Perfect Health Guide

The Teen who Refinanced his Mother's House and Car at 14

By: Danny Singh, B.S.B.I.M.
(Bachelor of Science in Business and Information Management)

Although Health Science is not my specialty, I always encourage individuals to avoid drugs and live healthy lifestyles because I do not want them to end their lives early like my father did due to alcohol. The book is meant to be a quick read.

The Whiz Kid's Perfect Health Guide

Profits support the Horizons for Homeless Children in Boston

Want to lower cholesterol levels? Want to increase your lifespan? Just want to read this book to kill time?

Well, congratulations because you have found the correct book. Please do not find the number of pages intimidating because the lessons contained within this book are meant to help consumers live the most healthy lifestyles ever by teaching them the significance of avoiding drugs, cutting down on fried foods, resolving conflicts in a peaceful manner, and learning how to treat diseases with tips presented on how to avoid contracting them in the first place. Danny Singh "financial whiz kid" refinanced his mother's house and car at 14 and has been doing seminars to educate students on how to detect diploma mill schools, save money by attending a community college, and repay their student loans with the least amount of interest and fees. Now he is focusing his attention on another issue. The Centers for Disease Control and Prevention has reported that heart disease and cancer are the 2 highest leading causes of death in America. In response to this epidemic, Danny advocates consumers avoiding dangerous substances, drugs, and breaking the addiction for the purpose of living the longest lives possible without worries.

Without needing expensive rehabilitation centers or fake drug treatment medicines advertised on the media, Danny will discuss strategies on how to resist taking drugs and focus more on consuming foods filled with vitamins, proteins, carbohydrates, and other nutrients. Such are recommended by the Food Guide Pyramid because they are vital for the overall well-being of a consumer. In addition to avoiding drugs, techniques will be presented on how consumers can incorporate daily exercise routines into their lifestyles while managing time for relationships with friends and family and completing tasks for work or school. As a result, consumers will be more likely to be mentally, emotionally, socially, and physically healthy.

No health book is complete without a discussion about the human body and its systems and Danny explains how they work together to fight infections, repair bone damages, and respond to hormonal changes especially during puberty. Regardless of the age of the consumer or their health conditions, this book will help anyone achieve all their health related goals. If the knowledge in this book does not improve your health then return or sell it! Nothing to lose but many ways to get healthy in The Whiz Kid's Perfect Health Guide!

Preview of Concepts (Some of Them at Least)
-Mental Health Disorders
-Social Relationships
-Personal Hygiene

-Dietary Guidelines
-Eating Disorders
-Organ Systems
-Communicable Diseases
-Pregnancy
-Environment Health

About the Author

With an Indian background, Danny Singh was the first in his family to be born and raised in Orlando, Florida; by his mother and grandparents. Danny's mother, Rita, purchased her own house in 2001, moved in with Danny. She began working longer hours at two jobs, so she could manage all the expenses. Due to the limited availability of Rita, Danny could not be fully dependent upon her.

For this reason, in 2003, Rita added Danny, as an authorized user, on her account and gave Danny his first credit card, at the age of 11; thus beginning his financial journey. Danny knew very little about credit cards and only used his credit card; to purchase food, supplies for school, necessities he needed, and gifts for his mom; during his younger years. He would always make sure his credit card was with him in his pocket. Danny admits to purchasing items he always desired, such as, Yu-Gi-Oh Cards, movies, comic books, Slurpee's at the gas station, and items kids would want. He loved the spending power of the credit card.

Unexpectedly, Rita started becoming increasingly busy on her jobs. She began calling Danny; asking him to open the mail and make sure the credit card bill was getting paid. She expressed; if the credit card bill was paid late, it would ruin her credit. Danny did not know what credit was, but he did not want to see his mother stress. While handling his academic responsibilities; he maintained her credit card, by signing online and using her checking account. As he began reading all of his mother's mail, although he could not understand everything; interest started provoking him as he began getting involved with other financial aspects of the household. Danny began reading the terms and conditions of the credit cards and the fine print, on the bills. This led him into reading more about credit on the Internet. He started asking his mother, grandfather, or the customer service credit managers; questions or misconceptions he had about credit.

Danny began wanting to handle the utility bills, mortgage, insurance, other credit cards (he was not using), and any other bill that his mother was expected to pay. Danny wanted his mother to give him full authorization, to all the companies; so they would release any account information to him, if needed. With this type of authorization, he would be permitted to make account changes, if needed, when calling customer service. Danny's mother was skeptical, at first, but trusted Danny; given the fact that he was never late on paying the credit card he was using.

Rita added Danny to all her accounts. They were discrete; about Danny's financial life. Danny has had many financial successes including: getting the annual fees removed from several of his mother's credit cards, refinancing the mortgage and car, getting over $1300 in interest refunded from a credit card company, having interest rates reduced on all loans, increasing the credit limits on accounts so his mother's credit scores could increase, and ensuring that no deposit accounts were becoming negative; at just 14 years of age.

Danny managed to get her car and house insurance costs reduced; while maintaining the same coverage. He removed a delinquency from his grandmother's credit report; which caused his grandmother to be denied credit. Danny was able to get his grandmother's credit application approved. When Rita's bank account information was stolen and numerous fraudulent charges occurred; Danny was able to get all the charges refunded. He also reported the phony business, to the Better Business Bureau and Complaint Board; so other consumers would not be scammed. Seminole County commissioner, Bob Dallari; Florida House District 33 representative, Jason Brodeur; Texas governor, Rick Perry; First Lady Anita Perry, Senator Marco Rubio, and several news stations recognized Danny; referring to him as a "financial whiz kid." In 2011, Danny graduated with honors from the International Baccalaureate program of University High School.

Danny has developed about eight years of financial experience, with many different financial institutions managing all the financial aspects of his mother's house and has never been late, even by a day, on several credit cards or any bill. Proudly, Danny is part of the Art & Phyllis Grindle Honors Institute, at the Seminole State College in Florida. Danny holds a Bachelor of Science in Business and Information Management. He hopes to earn an MBA and Ph.D., in Management, from the University of Central Florida. By doing financial seminars, running a financial tips website (www.facebook.com/studentsfinance), and his independent and non-profit credit advising agency; Danny encourages others that bankruptcy, debt settlements, being late, or not paying the bills are never solutions and success can only be achieved, with a powerful credit history. Danny hopes to one day work for a financial institution and continue sharing his financial passion. Helping others is what makes Danny's passion grow; so please contact him, using the Face Book page, if you need financial help.

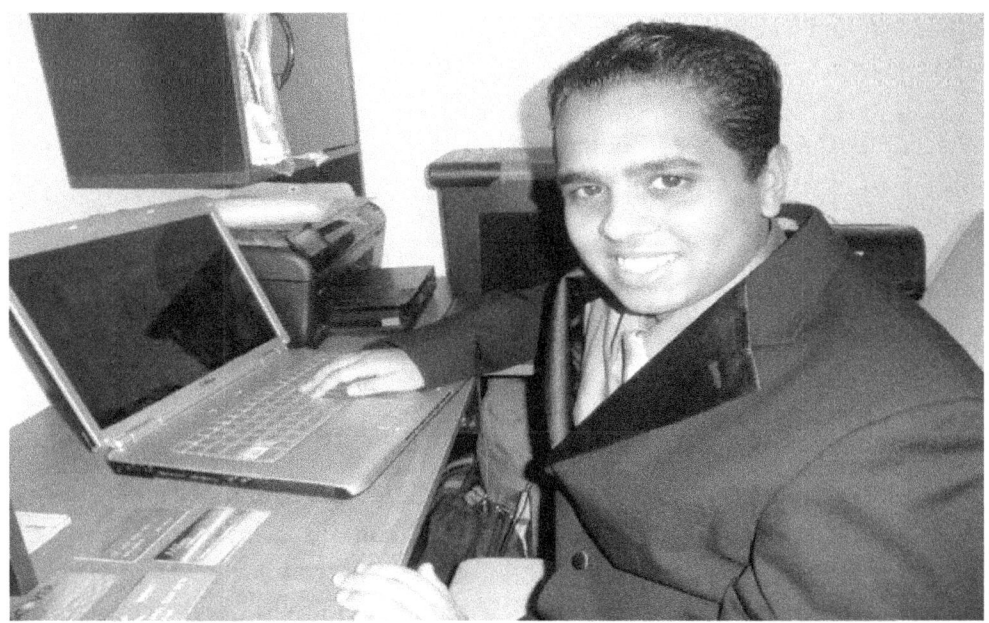

"Danny has demonstrated exceptional finance and accounting abilities and his accomplishments are impressive- especially considering his young age. His training has been invaluable. I am pleased to commend his excellence."
Rick Perry, Governor of Texas and First Lady Anita Perry

"I can say without reservation that Danny is a young man of impeccable character. Danny has taken a strong stand for his family as he began controlling the family finances. He is truly a unique individual who has had extremely different priorities."
Jason Brodeur, Florida State Representative, District 33

"Danny's extensive knowledge of credit and the banking industry that he shared with me greatly impressed me considering his young age. His financial talents are rare and he is with no doubt a very gifted individual with a bright future ahead."
Bob Dallari, Seminole County Commissioner, District 1

"Paying the bills and balancing a checkbook--all the task and responsibilities of being an adult. But one mom said she handed it all over to her son at just 11 years old."
Central Florida News 13

"Danny was a natural, a finance whiz kid. Soon, he was spending time reading the small print on each of his mom's credit card statements and every bill that came through. He started refinancing the ways banks work, how credit card companies calculate interest and what makes credit good."
East Orlando Sun

"Growing up Danny wanted to be a doctor. But that changed, the moment his mom gave him a new chore around the house. One that saved her thousands of dollars, and helped her son find a new path in life."
Dallas/Fort Worth WFAA-TV

"Danny accomplished the feat by negotiating with Bank of America was he was just 14 years old!"
Fox 35 News

"Feeling frustrated over finances? Need help managing a student loan? The Financial Whiz Kid may be able to help."
Seminole Chronicle

"You may have heard of Danny "Financial Whiz Kid" Singh. At the age of 11, the Orlando boy took over his mom's finances. By the age of 14, he had refinanced their home mortgage, persuaded banks to remove annual fees from his mom's credit cards and negotiated more than $1300 in refunds on interest and fees for her. His financial savvy attracted the attention of print and electronic media - and fellow high school students."
Seminole State College of Florida (Formerly, Seminole Community College)

Special Dedications

Ashish Yamdagni

A good friend of mine hoped to see more from me in the future and this encouraged me to write this new book. I cannot thank him enough for helping me stay motivated to share my knowledge with the world through the publications. This friend has my greatest respect because he always works beyond his limits and succeeds and I try to live up to his example. There have been times during high school; he was studying the entire night just to pass his one exam such as in Biology or Latin or complete a project to the highest level of perfection. Despite being a hard worker, he manages to have a humorous personality anyone can enjoy so if an individual needs a good laugh then they can always go to him. I proudly dedicate this book to Ashish Yamdagni.

Ashish is currently at the University of Miami doing the Pre-Med program. He also manages a business with his partner, Andrew Dang, called YDG Studios. The company helps customers with their digital and paper media needs. You can contact them through facebook at http://www.facebook.com/YDGStudios.

Steven Silvernail

I have made my share of mistakes in life but this person has helped me morph into a better person, realize my mistakes, and I vow to never make them again. His moral righteousness serves as a positive influence on my life and I cannot thank him enough for being him. I show my deepest respect to Steven Silvernail. He is studying to be a vet at the University of Central Florida. Some his courses are challenging and truthfully, I would fail at some of them but the challenge level never bothers him and he manages to surpass the expectations of the courses. Nothing brings him down and there is no doubt in my mind he will be successful. Just as how he has supported me in my endeavors, I hope to always support him.

Smit Vadvala

Throughout my junior and senior years at Seminole State College of Florida, I have had the honor of meeting, helping, and befriending Smit Vadvala. He is an immigrant from India and has inspired me in so many ways through his perseverance because he initially struggled to adjust to the lifestyle in the United States as well as to the school system. In addition, he has been providing for his sister and other family members by working extensive hours at a job. Regardless of the struggles, Smit has been passing several advanced college courses at Seminole State and has been maintaining a perfect grade point average. Smit hopes to earn the Bachelor of Science in Business and Information Management and later complete a Masters of Business Administration. Smit is a whiz when it comes to investing in stocks so a great deal of my financial knowledge has come from him. Smit, you have given me so much in the short time I have known you, thank you so much for it all. I hope we are friends forever and I could not have achieved the success that I did had it not been for you.

Endorsement

"Danny is originally a finance book author. However, under his caring and loving grandparents influence and by looking into their health matters, he started researching immensely into the health and medicine fields. This inspired to write this book which particularly deals with American people's health, lifestyle, and food habits and covers the teens' addiction of drugs and other issues. This book is really worth reading, bringing awareness, and it is for a good cause!"

-Smit Vadvala

Business and Information Management student at Seminole State College of Florida

Table of Contents

The Three Parts of Health

There are three parts of the Health Triangle that help individuals determine if they are overall healthy. The three parts are physical health, mental and emotional health, and social health.

Physical health involves taking care of the body. Individuals can be physically healthy by regularly exercising, eating a balanced diet, and getting plenty of sleep.

Mental and emotional health involves taking care of the mind. Individuals can be emotionally and mentally healthy by accepting themselves and expressing their feelings in a healthy manner. Individuals should also learn how to handle stress so they can avoid developing major depression.

Social health involves getting along with family members and people. Individuals can be socially healthy by keeping and making friends and learning to work well with others in groups despite having disagreements.

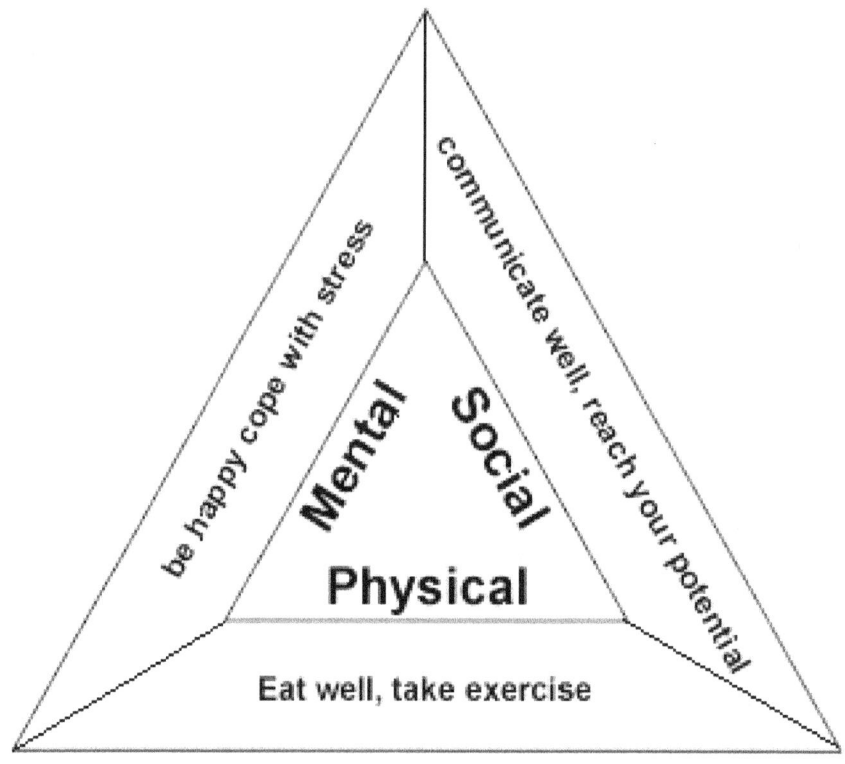

Source: http://www.islay.argyll-bute.sch.uk/courses/Biology%20Website%20files/int1/health/graphics/triangle.gif

Examples of Health Triangle Parts: Physical, Mental/Emotional, and Social

1. Going to a baseball game with friends- Social health.

2. Eating plenty of healthy foods- Physical health.

3. Hiding angry feelings- Mental and emotional health.

4. Helping friends with their problems- Social health.

5. Getting upset when a close individual passes away- Mental and emotional health.

6. An individual stays up late every night- Mental, emotional, and physical health.

7. An individual argues with another individual- Mental and emotional health. Arguing with friends can negatively affect the social health.

8. An individual thinks he or she is ugly- Mental and emotional health.

Controllable and Uncontrollable Factors of Health

Health Factors over which Individuals have Little or No Control

1. Hereditary is the passing on of traits from the parents to children as a result of the transmission of genes. Genes are strains of information such as hair color, eye color, and other characteristics that will create the new human.

2. The environment is the sum total of the surroundings.

3. The available health care, which is determined by the location of the individual where he or she lives and the rules established by the government.

Health Factors for which Individuals must be Responsible

1. Attitudes, which are the feelings and beliefs of an individual. A positive attitude means a healthier life.

2. Lifestyle factors, which are life-related habits. Healthy habits can include exercising, eating healthy foods, and spending time with good friends. Unhealthy habits can include taking risks, the usage of drugs, and having a low self-concept.

3. Individuals should get the best education possible to best improve their health conditions. Some individuals ignorantly do unhealthy habits such as smoking and they are not aware of the harm they are causing to their bodies.

Habits of Healthy People

1. Get regular exercise such as running or swimming.

2. Avoid using tobacco, alcohol, and/or drugs.

3. Get at least eight hours of sleep each night.

4. Practice good grooming habits. Such can include brushing and flossing their teeth each day.

5. Express feelings in appropriate ways.

6. Work well in groups.

7. Do not take unnecessary chances on risks.

8. Stay informed about health-related issues.

9. Have regular medical and dental checkups.

10. Use seat belts when they are riding in an automobile.

11. Take time to relax when they are feeling stress.

12. Think positively and have an upbeat outlook.

Mental and Emotional Health

Mental and emotional health is the ability of the individual to accept and like themselves and others. To be mentally and emotionally healthy, an individual must adapt and cope with their emotions and feelings, handle problems, conflicts, and changes within their lives.

How to be Mentally and Emotionally Healthy

1. An individual sees themselves and life mostly in positive ways.

2. An individual faces challenges with confidence and determination.

3. An individual motivates and encourages themselves to achieve long-term goals.

4. An individual recognizes and manages their feelings.

5. An individual focuses on their strengths.

6. An individual accepts honest criticisms and learns from their mistakes in order to improve upon themselves.

How to be Emotionally Healthy

Emotional needs are the needs that affect the feelings and sense of well-being.

The basic emotional needs of an individual include

1. The need to feel worthwhile is to feel that an individual is making a contribution.

2. The need to love and be loved is to feel special and to make others feel special.

3. The need to belong is to feel that an individual is part of a group.

An individual should satisfy their emotional needs in healthy ways and engage in healthy behavior.

A way to avoid unhealthy behavior is to

Practice abstinence, which is refusing to participate in unsafe behaviors. Such behaviors can include sex, using drugs, or committing a crime.

Stand up to pressure by using refusal skills.

One way to say no effectively is to look at the individual firmly and say "no" with confidence.

Stress

Stress is the response of the individual to changes of any type around them such as different people, a different home, or different living conditions. When the body feels stress then the heart beats faster.

An object, event, person, or place that triggers stress is a stressor. Adrenaline is a type of hormone that prepares the body to respond to stress and this is part of the reason why the heart beats faster.

There are two types of stress.

Positive Stress
Feelings: Challenged, excited, alert, and focused.

An example of an incident that might create positive stress is playing on a sports team.

Negative Stress
Feelings: Disappointed, angry, frustrated, sadness, helpless, loneliness, and confused.

An example of an incident that might create negative stress is arguing with a friend. Other examples of negative stress can include failing grades, bullies, getting sick, and other people fighting whom have a relationship with the individual.

How the Body Responds to Stress

Physical Fatigue
Cause: Vigorous activity.

Solution: Relaxing.

Emotional Fatigue (Tiredness)
Cause: Negative stress, worrying, and feelings of sadness.

Solution: Removing the source of stress or learning how to manage it.

Ways to Reduce Stress

1. Plan ahead and be proactive. An example of being proactive can be having an umbrella in the car in the event that it rains.

2. Set priorities.

3. Redirect the energy.

4. Talk to a good friend or parent.

5. Relax.

Conflict

A conflict is a problem in a relationship of some type. An example of a conflict can be a disagreement between people with opposing viewpoints.

Four Steps to Prevent Conflict
1. Practice tolerance.
2. Individuals should express their thoughts and feelings freely provided that they do not hurt the feelings of other individuals. This is because hurting others can create more conflict.
3. Walk away.
4. "Deflate" the situation.

Three Ways to Resolve Conflict

A. Make a compromise, which means to make an agreement with an individual in which each person, gives up something. This is done for the purpose of reaching a solution that satisfies everyone involved with the conflict.

B. Communicate
-Choose the right time and place to speak to the individual.
-Stick to the point.
-Stay clam.
-Choose words carefully.
-Show respect.
-Listen.

C. Call in a peer mediator such as a close teacher or friend
-Establish neutrality.
-Set the ground rules.
-Listen to all sides respectfully.
-Search for possible solutions.
-Do not give up.

Abuse- No Individual Should Tolerate

Abuse is the emotional, mental, and physical mistreatment of an individual.

Types of Abuse

*In some cases, multiple types of abuse occur.

Physical abuse

When an individual uses some means to physically inflict harm on another individual. For example, if a parent beats their child everyday then this is considered physical abuse.

Emotional or mental abuse

Emotional or mental abuse is taking place when an individual often says unpleasant or hurtful comments to another individual. This can possibly cause the listener to think badly of themselves. An example of such abuse can be when a parent calls their child derogatory names or uses curse words when speaking to them.

Sexual abuse

When an individual inappropriately touches another individual, makes inappropriate sexual comments, or forcefully has sex with them. For example, incest is when a family member rapes or molests another family member and this is a type of sexual abuse.

Neglect

The individual fails to properly care for another individual. An example of neglect can be if a mother never feeds food to her baby.

Causes of Abuse

There are many causes behind why an individual abuses another individual. Regardless of the cause, it is unethical and can lead to the death of the individual being abused.

-If an individual has a mental disease of any type.
-If an individual is using drugs or powerful substances.
-If an individual has undergone a divorce or other painful experience.
-If an individual was abused themselves.
-If an individual often gets angry and does not know how to manage their anger in a healthy manner.

Signs of Abuse

If an individual knows of another individual being abused then they should report it immediately to a local police station, family member of the individual with whom they have a good relationship, or a school guidance counselor. In doing so, the individual is saving the life of the individual who is being abused. Individuals can tell if a person is being abused by paying attention to the signs below.

-If an individual is often absent from school or their job.
-If the performance of the individual is poor with school or their job.
-If the individual often gets angry, violent, or has mood swings for minor reasons.
-If the individual is often sad, tired, and/or upset.
-If the individual looks malnourished or their appearance is poor such as if they are always wearing dirty clothes.
-If the individual has the inability to communicate.

Sources of Help

-Police department.
-Doctors.
-Crisis hotlines.
-Family counseling centers or school counselors.
-Family violence shelters.
-Support groups.

Emotional Expression

Exercising may help an individual express their feelings such as happiness, anger, or sadness. During the teen years, hormones may cause rapid physical changes in the body.

Creating a project may help an individual express their feelings or emotions.

Being alone may give an individual the opportunity to think about why an individual feels the way that they do so.

Communication is the exchange of the thoughts and feelings between 2 or more people.

Hormones are special chemicals, produced by glands that regulate many functions of the body. Some hormones may causes changes with the mood of an individual. This may affect their communication with others.

Communicating, or talking to others, may help an individual understand their feelings.

Types of Communication
-Words.
-Facial expressions.
-Gestures.
-Posture.
-Overall body language.

Six Rules to Follow when Speaking
1. An individual should think before they speak.
2. An individual should be honest without being hurtful.
3. Do not do all the talking. Give the other individual an opportunity to speak out of respect.
4. Individuals should be aware of their listeners.
5. Send the same message verbally and non-verbally.
6. Be specific.

Six Rules to Follow when Listening
1. Ask questions.
2. Try not to interrupt the individual.
3. Concentrate.
4. Keep an open mind.
5. Paraphrase what the individual says to show respect and understanding.
6. Look and sound like a listener. For example, an individual who is listening should not be looking at other places besides the person with whom they are communicating.

Goal Setting Skills

A goal is what an individual hopes to accomplish or achieve during a certain time. For this reason, the individual will work for satisfying the goal. There are 2 types of goals, which are long-term goals and short-term goals. The names of the 2 types of goals are self-explanatory. A long-term goal can take months or years to complete such as earning a college degree. In contrast, a short-term goal only takes a couple days or weeks. An example of a short-term goal can be winning a basketball game that will take place tomorrow. When trying to achieve any type of goal, an individual should develop an action plan.

Parts of an Action Plan

1. Identify a goal.

2. Indicate the actions needed to achieve the goal.

3. Identify sources of help and support to achieve the goal.

4. Establish a time period by the end of which the goal will be achieved.

5. Set up checkpoints at which the individual will evaluate how much progress they have made in achieving the goal.

6. Establish a reward that the individual will receive when they have achieved the goal.

7. Indicate any extra benefits that may result from achieving the goal.

Six Stages of Decision Making

Step 1

State the situation. The individual should ask themselves how the problem developed.

Step 2

List the options. Think of many ways to solve the problem.

Step 3

Weigh the possible outcomes. Individuals should think of all the pros and cons of each possible decision.

Step 4

Individuals should consider their values when making a decision. They should not make a decision that goes against their values.

Step 5

Individuals should make a decision and act. Decide which option is best for the people involved and act on that choice.

Step 6

Evaluate the decision. Decide whether the solution worked and if the outcome was in the overall favor of the individual.

Traits of Good Character

Character is the way in which a person thinks, feels, and acts towards themselves and others. Character involves understanding, caring about, and acting upon certain values. Values are the beliefs an individual uses to guide themselves throughout their life. A character trait is a quality that demonstrates how a person thinks, feels, and behaves.

Primary Traits of Good Character

Trustworthiness

Respect

Responsibility

Citizenship

Fairness

Caring

Kindness

Self-Concept

The self-concept of an individual is how he or she views themselves.

If it is a negative self-concept then an individual focuses mostly on their flaws.

If it is a positive self-concept then an individual focuses mostly on their strengths.

The self-esteem of an individual is the way he or she feel about themselves.

To raise self-esteem, an individual needs to focus on their strengths, accept constructive criticism, and learn as well as improve from their mistakes.

Mental Health Disorders

Anxiety Disorders
Mental disorders (problems) that are influenced by extreme feelings, anxiety, or fear.

Examples: General anxiety disorder, obsessive-compulsive disorder, phobia, panic structured feelings and disorder.

Reactions, signs, and symptoms
Each anxiety disorder has a different set of symptoms. The common relation between most anxiety disorders is that they may cause an individual to have mood swings and/or feel insecure.

Mood Disorders
When an individual experiences extreme or prolonged emotions or mood changes that they cannot control.

Examples: Major depression or manic-compulsive (sometimes called the bipolar disorder).

Reactions, Signs, and Symptoms
The individual may over exaggerate the severity of their problems, they may get upset easily, and they may have mood swings. They may start taking drugs of some type to relax themselves from the mood disorder.

Schizophrenia
A severe mental disorder in which people lose contact with reality.

Reactions, signs, and symptoms
Hallucinations, delusions, faulty beliefs, separation from what is really happening, and behaving in unusual ways.

Treatment for Mental Health Disorders

Methods of Therapy for Mental Health Problems

Talk therapy includes a variety of counseling methods.

Biological therapy uses drug treatments as medication.

The goal of all treatment methods for mental health problems is to help the person change so that they can manage their problems better, feel less stress, and live a healthier life.

Source of Help for Mental and Emotional Problems

1. Talk to a parent or other family member.

2. Clergy member.

3. Teacher or school counselor.

4. Family counselor.

5. School nurse.

6. Psychologist.

7. Psychiatrist.

Social Relationships

1. Responsible Dating
-Showing respect for others.
-Being trustworthy.
-Thinking about the consequences of their actions.

2. Emotional Maturity
-Being prepared to make a marriage work.
-Having plans for reaching goals.
-Understand the needs of others such as the children and spouse.
-At first, put the needs of others first especially the children because they are dependent on their parents.

3. Socializing
-Communicating with other people preferably in a healthy manner.
-Getting along with other people.
-Working out differences of opinions and respecting ideas.

4. Divorce
-Marriage not working.
-Breakup of a family.
-Possibility of a new and happier family.
*Divorce should be the absolute last option in relationships because a marriage is sacred. As a personal opinion, a divorce disrespects a marriage.

5. Failure of Teen Marriages
-Emotional immaturity.
-Not enough money.
-Too young to be parents and thus, too stressful.

6. Marriage Commitment
-Pledging to respect the needs of others.
-Promising to make the relationship stronger and being authentic.
-An individual sharing themselves with another person.

7. Group Dating
-Getting used to being with people in a social situation.
-Avoiding the pressure to break apart.
-Going out with friends and/or classmates of both genders.

Friendship and Qualities of Good Friends

Friendship is considered a special type of relationship between people who enjoy the presence of each other and feel good.

Reasons for Making and Keeping Friends
1. Similar interests.
2. Similar values.
3. Personal qualities.
4. Same school or neighborhood.

Peer pressure is when one friend influences another friend to do a certain act. Good friends do not give individuals negative peer pressure such as to do drugs, break the law, or participate in an activity that is harmful to themselves and/or others. They give positive peer pressure to individuals. The positive peer pressure will help the individual finish tasks such as finish writing a book, eat healthy, exercise, and participate in activities that are beneficial.

Qualities of Good Friends

Trustworthy: Believe what an individual says is truthful. This means no information is being hidden or changed and the individual has no bad motives.

Reliable: Can rely on an individual to perform a task or do a favor.

Empathetic: Can relate to the problems of an individual or emotionally connect with them and show understanding of their feelings.

Caring: Be considerate and show concern when an individual is facing trouble of some type.

Respectful: Be polite to the decisions, ideas, and opinions of individuals.

Tips for Making Friends

1. Start a conversation with individuals at school, work, or church. Individuals should try to socialize with other individuals with whom they may have similar interests.

2. Individuals should join clubs, groups, or organizations to meet new people and possibly befriend them.

3. Individuals should offer to help others.

4. If invited, individuals should join group hangouts such as if a group of people plan to see a movie.

5. Individuals should be polite when making a first impression on new people.

6. Individuals should try socializing with their peers, who are people close to their age group.

Families

Five Types of Families

1. Nuclear family: Usually 2 parents, which are mom and dad, and children.

2. Couple family: A married couple with no children.

3. Single-parent family: Children with either a mom or dad.

4. Extended family: Nuclear or single parent family plus other relatives such as uncles, aunties, cousins, or grandparents.

5. Blended family: Divorced individuals from previous marriages marry each other and they have children from the previous marriages.

Four Recent Changes in Families

1. Single-parent families from result from a divorce.

2. The mother may work outside the home.

3. Smaller families.

4. Mobile families.

Four Ways to have a Healthy Family

1. Communicate.

2. Spend time together.

3. Keep traditions.

4. Be flexible.

Family Problems

1. Physical abuse.

2. Emotional abuse.

3. Sexual abuse.

4. Neglect.

Five Places to Turn for Help

1. Family counseling.

2. Crisis hot lines.

3. Youth services.

4. Shelters.

5. Support and self-help groups.

Myths and Facts about the Family Life

1. All families consist of a father, mother, and children.
Myth: There are single-parent families, extended families, families with just non-blood relatives, and possibly other family types too depending upon their customs and cultures.

2. The way an individual feels about themselves affects their decisions.
Fact: Individuals feeling sad, depressed, or upset may take drugs to make themselves feel better. They may possibly have sex to boost their confidence. This is not wise because these bad decisions can have serious health consequences.

3. Peer pressure is always bad.
Myth: Peer pressure can be good or bad. For example, if a friend encourages an individual to have sex then this is considered bad peer pressure. This is because the friend is influencing the individual to make a very bad decision and the individual could get infected with some type of sexually transmitted disease such as HIV. An example of good peer pressure can be encouraging an individual to study for an exam. This is positive influence that will result in success for the individual.

4. An abused child always becomes an abusive parent.
Myth: It is possible for an abused child to one day become a loving parent. The child may learn from the bad experiences with their parents. This may motivate the child to become the best parent possible towards their children. However, it is also possible the abusive treatment instilled violent tendencies within the child and these tendencies may start reflecting increasingly as they become an adult. For this problem, an adult who was abused as a child can get special counseling so the adult is not abusive towards their children and continues the cycle. This is because the possibility rises that the children will become abusive towards the grandchildren of their abusive parents.

5. Alcohol and drug abuse can interfere with making the right decisions.
Fact: Drugs and alcohol have chemicals that can cause an individual to have changes with their behavior. This is because the chemicals of alcohol and drugs cause the body to have certain reactions that influence the functions of the body systems such as the endocrine system. Hormones may secrete chemicals that could cause the individual to feel tense, sad, angry, or another mood. For example, if an individual drinks alcohol, their heart rate may increase, and the individual may participate in some type of dangerous activity. An example of a dangerous activity is driving over the speed limit.

6. During puberty, boys and girls can become parents.
Fact: Puberty allows for the body to physically mature so individuals are capable of having children. However, mentally and emotionally, it is unlikely young individuals are

ready to have kids. As a personal recommendation, individuals should only have kids after getting married. This is because without marriage, if one of the partners leaves then the other partner can only get child support and not alimony. This money will support the well-being of the children. Child support alone is usually not enough money to live a decent lifestyle. Therefore, alimony is also needed by the single parent.

7. One purpose of the menstrual cycle is to rid the body of an unfertilized egg.
Fact: This is a natural bodily process of all women.

8. If a girl has never had a period, she cannot get pregnant.
Myth: It is possible for a girl who has never had a period to get pregnant. Not having a period means for whatever reason, the body of the girl is taking a long time to release the blood and other material from the womb. Girls can get more advice from their doctors about why they are not having periods.

9. Once an individual gets HIV then they will always have it.
Fact: Unfortunately, there is no cure for HIV or vaccine. It is a chronic disease. For this reason, individuals should never have sex unless they are in a committed relationship. They are very confident their partner is not having sexual relationships with other people. Besides sex, there are other means through which HIV can be transmitted.

10. HIV cannot be transmitted from an infected mother to her unborn child.
Myth: Unfortunately, it is possible for the infected mother and her child to have blood-to-blood contact when she is giving birth. This will cause the baby to get HIV.

11. STDs (Sexually Transmitted Diseases) are communicable diseases.
Fact: Individuals who have STDs can transmit them to their partners through sexual contact or any type of blood-to-blood contact.

12. Abstinence is the only 100% effective treatment to prevent pregnancy.
Fact: Unmarried individuals should not have sex because it can ruin their lives especially if they become pregnant. Women may have to drop out of school. This is to lower the likelihood of any fatal occurrence happening to their child during the development inside them.

Childhood and Adolescence

Puberty is the time when an individual begins to develop certain physical traits of the adults of their gender.

During adolescence, an individual develops their own set of values.

Four Stages of Growth Leading to Adulthood

1. The first year of the life of a child is called infancy.

2. Children between the ages of one and three are called toddlers.

3. Children aged three to five are usually called preschoolers.

4. The period between childhood and adulthood is adolescence.

Physical Changes

Five changes that occur in both boys and girls are

1. Acne (skin aliment).

2. Growth spurt.

3. Facial bone structure.

4. Pubic hair.

5. Underarm hair.

6. Increase in perspiration.

Emotional and Mental Changes

- Changes in moods are usually caused by hormones.

- Social Changes

- During adolescence, the relationships with parents, friends, and families change.

Saving a Marriage from Divorce

1. Individuals should not talk to their spouses disrespectfully or use curse words regardless of how upset they are for whatever reasons. Disrespectful talking makes both individuals very upset and raises the likelihood of the marriage failing.

2. Individuals should positively communicate with their spouse about their expectations and needs. They should be honest with their spouse about what their spouse does that makes them upset and they kindly want to see a change.

3. Individuals should not tell other family members, friends, or children about the problems within the marriage. If individuals are greatly sad and need a close friend with whom to talk about the issues then they should do so. However, they still should not tell everyone about the relationship issues. This is because it is possible that family members or friends may cause more distrust to develop between the 2 spouses.

4. Individuals should be honest about the mistakes they have made and the steps they will take to rectify them. If they need help to stop making the mistakes then they need to seek the appropriate help. For example, if a spouse is cheating on their spouse then personally, this is considered a sin and the spouse needs to be honest about it. The 2 spouses should get a marriage or relationship counselor. However, if the spouse is continuing to be unfaithful then a divorce is highly encouraged. This is because usually spouses who cheat have low character and it is a bad habit that they will not change. Spouses should not have sexual relationships with spouses who have cheated on them until they both have had counseling. Spouses who have cheated should get a medical checkup on themselves to make sure they do not have any sexually transmitted diseases. In doing so, they prevent the chances of passing on STDs to their spouse. They should not make excuses to hide their mistakes and their spouses should not be easily convinced their spouses have truly reformed and will no longer make the same mistakes. Cheating is a serious issue.

5. If possible, spouses can occasionally ask their parents to watch over the children and they can spend time alone for the purpose of getting emotionally close. Provided they both have not cheated, the 2 spouses should be open to the idea of having sexual intercourse. This is because it can serve as a means of strengthening the love and trust.

6. Regardless of the problems within the marriage, spouses should not be romantic with other individuals or consider dating others. This may cause more problems and distrust.

7. Both spouses should discuss with each other the reasons why they fell in love and decided to get married. They should embrace the reasons and make each other realize how much they appreciate the individual. If one or more of the spouses still feel trapped within the marriage then divorce or separation are the best options.

Being a Consumer

A consumer is any individual who buys services or goods.

How to Be a Wise Consumer

Use money wisely.

Buy useful goods and services.

Buy safe goods and services.

Know what to do if an individual has a consumer problem.

Why Be a Wise Consumer?

To promote and protect the health of an individual.

To save time and money.

To build self-confidence.

To protect their rights.

Safety Conscious

Being safety conscious means being aware that safety is always important. For this reason, individuals must act safely and make wise decisions.

Resist peer pressure.

An individual should concentrate on what they are doing and not make hasty decisions.

An individual should know their limits and be prepared for dangers or risks.

How to Avoid Scams

When reading advertisements, consumers must watch out for certain factors.

1. Quackery, which means selling worthless products or services by making false claims or over exaggerations.

2. Messages that sound too good to be true.

3. Products sold through these three services:

A. An unfamiliar mail source.

B. Cable and satellite television shows.

C. People who come to the house or location of the individual.

If the product disappoints the individual then he or she may not be able to get their money returned.

When comparing products, individuals should focus on certain factors.

1. Price
Think: How much can I afford to pay?

2. Benefits or features
Think: Does one brand offer benefits that another brand does not?

3. Reputation
Think: Do I know anyone who uses and likes this brand?

4. Warranty
Think: Will I get my money back if the product does not work as claimed?

When comparing stores and competitors, consumers should focus on these factors.

1. Convenience
Think: Will going to the store waste time and money especially on gas?

2. Return policies

Think: Can an individual get their money back or refunded. Will the store only give credit? Store credit means the individual can buy items only from the particular store. The amount of store credit they will receive depends upon how much money they paid for the item that they are returning to the store.

3. Sales and discounts.
Think: Does one store often lower its prices on certain products?

4. Sales staff and workers
Think: Are the clerks helpful?

Advertising Techniques: Seek the Hidden Message

In order for individuals to be healthy, they must avoid getting fooled by advertisers selling unhealthy products such as fried foods and drugs. Consumers who purchase unhealthy products not only damage their health but also damage their financial conditions. This could one day lead to negative stress as individuals become closer towards the age of retirement. Below are some of the techniques advertisers are using to attract consumers.

Bandwagon: Everyone purchases the item or service so this should serve as a sufficient reason for the individual to purchase the same item or service.

Testimonial: A famous individual that is credible and admirable uses the item or service. For this reason, the individual should use the same item or service.

Glamour or Sexual Appeal: Individuals in the advertisement are extremely good-looking and sexy. The idea is that if an individual buys the product then they will be similarly sexy and glamorous in appearance.

Snob Appeal: The advertisement stresses that the product is the best and is costly. The idea is that the product is awesome because it is expensive. This suggests the product is of high quality. If an individual can afford the product then they have good taste and are likely rich.

Dreams and Insecurities: Tobacco advertisers use different strategies to attract individuals. Cigarette advertisements geared to young women play on the idea of being "liberated" and in control – while at the same time playing on insecurities about the body image. Brands geared towards women often have words like "slim" or "slender" in the product name, or use extremely thin models in their advertisements. Cigarette advertisements geared to young men use rugged, independent, masculine-looking models, such as the classical image of the Marlboro Man. These models are usually shown participating in sports or outdoor activities, or surrounded by attractive women.

Lifestyle: Using this product or service will help individuals find friends and have fun. Cigarette firms have long used "pictures of health" in cigarette advertisements to promote smoking as an acceptable and healthy lifestyle. These advertisements want for consumers to associate smoking with outdoor sports and recreational activities such as tennis, bicycling, sailing, and horseback riding.

Popularity Appeal: Using this product or service will make the individual popular with other individuals.

Comparison: The organization compares its product directly with another product, saying it is better. (One is better or not as harmful as another).

Wit and Humor: People are attracted to advertisements that are funny. It makes an individual think of happy thoughts when they think about the product.

Regular Folks: People "just like you," are shown using this product. The idea is that the individual will trust these people because they are like them. The individual will likely think of them as peers instead of actors or models.

Leaving Out Facts: Telling the good side of something and leaving out the bad side.

Personal Hygiene

Personal hygiene: A routine of personal care that keeps the whole body clean, healthy, and fresh. Good hygiene helps an individual look and feel their best. It also affects how they feel about themselves and how others feel about them.

Nutrition: Eat properly using the Food Guide Pyramid and drink 6 to 8 glasses of water everyday.

Exercise: Individuals should do physical activities such as running at least 3 times per week to avoid becoming overweight.

Sleep: Individuals should sleep about 6 to 9 hours every night.

Ears
Wash them daily, especially behind the ears; see a doctor for wax build up.

Hands
Wash often before touching food, after using the toilet, and use gloves when giving first aid.

Hair
Brush daily, wash regularly (everyday of every other day), rinse brushes and combs, watch for dandruffs, hair losses, and sores.

Skin
Bathe and shower everyday, use soap and a washcloth and poof, use deodorants or antiperspirants, wear clean underwear, socks, and clothes, deal with skin problems.

Girls: Replace pads and tampons often.

Teeth
Brush twice a day, floss teeth, and get regular checkups at least once a year.

Feet
Wash feet daily and dry well. Use powder to soften corns and calluses (patches of thickened skin) and to prevent odor, cut nails.

Tooth Decay: An Ugly Process

Tooth decay is when a tooth in the mouth becomes bad, it may become less white, and it may cause the individual to feel pain all the time or when they eat food. For this reason, individuals must see the dentist periodically and brush twice a day. If they do not have dental insurance, they can often find coupons in the newspaper or in the mail for affordable checkup and cleaning prices.

Tooth Decay Steps

1. Air, food, and bacteria surround the tooth.

2. Bacteria, food particles, and salvia form plaque on the tooth.

3. The plaque interacts with sugars from the food and this creates acid.

4. If the plaque is not removed immediately then it may harden into tartar. Tartar will cause the overall conditions of the teeth to become worse, the individual may experience more pain, and it will become more expensive for them to afford proper dental treatment.

5. Acid under the plaque or tartar eats a cavity in the tooth enamel.

6. Decay spreads to the dentin.

7. Decay spreads to the pulp, where it exposes a nerve.

8. If the decay is not stopped, pus collects around the tooth and creates an abscess. This looks very gross.

No Dental Insurance?

It is important to see a dentist regularly for checkups and cleaning of the teeth. If an individual does not have dental insurance then they should look in the newspaper, mail, and internet to seek coupons or specials offered by local dentists.

Parts of the Skin

Epidermis
Outermost layer of skin that contains several layers of cells including cells in the deepest part that produce melanin.

Dermis
Thick inner layer of skin that contains blood vessels, nerve endings, hair follicles, and oil as well as sweat glands.

Subcutaneous Layer
This is the layer below the dermis that contains the fat cells and connects the skin to the bones and muscles.

Human Hair

Each strand of the human hair has three layers. The outer layer is sometimes called the cuticle and it is composed of several scales similar to the skin of a fish. If the scales are smooth then the hair usually looks glossy. If the scales are damaged or rough then the hair looks dull.

The middle layer is sometimes called the cortex and it consists of strong and elastic cells. These cells contain a substance called melanin, which colors the hair.

The innermost layer of the hair is mostly spongy tissue.

Oily sebums from the sebaceous glands make the hair look glossy as well as supple. This affects how greasy or dry the hair is of an individual.

The shape of the pit, sometimes called the follicle, which each hair grows from, determines how curly or straight each hair will be in appearance.

Each hair is attached to a muscle and can contract, which makes the hairs stand on the end. This can trap warmth between the hairs when an individual feels cold.

Human Hair Problems

Dandruff is a build up of dead skin cells stuck together with sebum on the scalp. Dandruff is not considered to be an infection and does not respond to the antiseptic in medicated shampoos. If an individual has dandruff then it is recommended that they wash their hair often and gently use mild shampoo. Individuals need to be careful of anti-dandruff shampoos because they may irritate the scalp. For this reason, individuals who are not sure how to deal with dandruff should consult with a doctor.

Lice are little insects that lay eggs and stick them to the scalp. The eggs are very difficult to get removed. Usually a symptom of having lice is that an individual will scratch their head often. Lice are very contagious and must be treated quickly. Some retail stores may sell certain lotions that can be used to kill the eggs of the lice.

Problems with the Human Eye

Farsightedness

Visual images come to a focus behind the retina.

Close objects to appear blurred.

Nearsightedness

Visual images come to a focus before they reach the retina.

This causes the distant objects to appear blurred.

Astigmatism

Visual images do not meet at a single point in the eye.

Images appear to be distorted or blurred.

Measuring Age

Age is measured in 3 ways.

-Chronological age: The number of the most recent birthday.

-Biological age: How well various body parts work.

-Social age: The lifestyle and habits of an individual.

Old age is more rewarding for people who

-Have dealt with changes effectively.

-Maintain contact with family and friends.

-Get involved with younger people.

Stages of Dying

Stages of Dying

1. Denial

2. Anger

3. Bargaining

4. Depression

5. Acceptance

Stages of Grief

1. Shock

2. Anger

3. Yearning

4. Depression

5. Moving on

Coping Strategies
For dealing with the death of a loved individual

1. Remembering good qualities about the person.

2. Not running away from the feelings.

3. Sharing feelings with other individuals.

4. Joining a support group.

Health Care System

Medicaid and Medicare are two government health care programs for people who are having a major financial hardship or over 65 years of age.

A family doctor provides basic health care for people of all ages.

A specialist is a doctor who is trained to handle a particular health problem.

Ophthalmologist: Treats diseases of the eyes.

Pediatrician: Treats children.

Urologist: Treats problems of the urinary system.

Dermatologist: Treats skin conditions and diseases.

Cardiologist: Treats heart problems.

Allergist: Treats Asthma, hay fever, and other allergies.

Otolaryngologist: Treats the ear, nose, and throat.

Orthopedist: Treats broken bones.

All states and most local governments have health departments. An example of such a department is the Department of Sanitation or Water.

Many people buy health insurance to help pay for the high costs of health care.

A hospice is a medical center for dying patients and it is financially supported by social welfare.

A health maintenance organization (HMO) is a group of health care providers that provides health care for its members.

Health Organizations
-National Multiple Sclerosis Society.
-American Diabetes Association.
-American Heart Association.
-Alzheimer's Association.

Dietary Guidelines

1. Individuals should eat a variety of foods using the Food Pyramid, which can be found on http://kidshealth.org/kid/stay_healthy/food/pyramid.html. This is because different foods give them different types of energy and such is vital for healthy living.

2. Individuals should stay at a healthy body weight because being overweight causes the body to work harder and this puts more stress on the heart. For this reason, being overweight can cause heart disease, high blood pressure (hypertension), diabetes, cancer, and stroke. The condition of being overweight often causes individuals to lack energy and this makes it harder for the human body to fight off illnesses.

3. Individuals must be careful of fat. Only a tablespoon of fat is needed every day. Excessive fat leads to becoming overweight. This can cause several heart problems.

4. Fiber is an ideal nutrient for the body. Fiber speeds food as it goes through the digestive system. Fiber can be found in foods such as fruits, vegetables, and grains. Fiber can help reduce the risk of heart disease and certain types of cancer when individuals get older.

5. Individuals should be careful of how much sugary foods they consume because usually, sugary foods have very few vitamins and minerals. As a healthy alternative to wanting a sweet food, individuals can eat the natural sugar. This is found in fruits such as bananas and mangoes. In eating these fruits, individuals will be able to get some vitamins, fiber, and minerals along with their satisfied desire of wanting a sweet fruit.

6. Individuals only need a teaspoon of salt each day. Consuming excessive amounts of salt can cause high blood pressure and the stress on the circulatory system can lead to a heart attack.

7. Individuals should avoid drinking alcohol and beer because these substances gradually destroy the tissues (groups of living cells) in the brain and liver. When the cells are destroyed then more cells are not created. For this reason, alcohol and beer increases the likelihood of an individual developing some type of cancer.

How to Eat

Remember that nothing in excess is good for individuals, meaning too much of any substance or food is not healthy.

Water is really healthy for individuals, and unfortunately, many people do not drink enough water. Individuals should try to drink about six to eight glasses of water each day. However, individuals should not force themselves to drink water if they are not thirsty.

Individuals should use their thirst mechanism similar to their breathing mechanism, sleep mechanism, and hunger mechanism. If an individual is thirsty then they should drink water.

How to Feed the Stomach

The true feeling of hunger is when an individual feels a little burning, empty, and hollow sensation that occurs several hours after the individual last ate. Rumbles in the lower intestine (below the waistline) are not stomach hunger signs. They are just digestion noises. If individuals are not sure if they are really hungry then they should wait a little longer. It feels great while individuals are waiting. If an individual is truly hungry, the hunger feeling will come back within about 45 minutes.

The blood sugar level of the individual is raised after they eat. The blood sugar level drops when the individual has not consumed food in a while. When the blood sugar level drops, the brain sends a message to the stomach to produce hydrochloric acid which produces the hunger pangs (empty, hollow, burning, hunger feelings). It is similar to when the fuel gauge in an automobile points to "E" for empty. However, individuals are not truly on empty, because their body has an excess of stored fuel in their body fuel.

When an individual reaches the hunger stage but are not able to get to food for ten to twenty minutes, the body pulls a meal from the stored fuel (stored body fat) and places it in the bloodstream. The hunger growls go away and the individual has fuel on which they function.

Individuals should not ignore true hunger (stomach growls). If an individual does then doing so is considered as bad a habit as overeating when the body tells the individual to stop eating because they are full or in other words, satisfied. Individuals should listen to what their body is telling them to do and do it.

If an individual wants to drink beverages that have sugar in them with the meals then this is considered normal. However, if an individual is just having a drink, they are recommended to try non-caloric drinks such as water. If an individual drinks sugared drinks, the blood sugar levels will not lower and the stomach will not growl or feel hungry. An individual will have a harder time knowing when they are hungry. This may lead to becoming unhealthy.

When eating, individuals should sip their drink between bites so that they can taste and enjoy the food more easily for the purpose of feeling satisfied. This feeling makes it less likely that the individual will overeat, which can lead to becoming fat.

When an individual eats then they should rate each food. First, individuals should eat the foods that they like the most because they are not sure when they will feel full or satisfied. It is easier to stop eating the least-favorite foods on their plate than the most-favorite foods. Dissect the food on their plate so that the best bites are in the stomach. Individuals should leave dessert for last, and save room for it. (Please do not wait until you are full and then eat dessert).

In America, restaurant portions of food are much larger than we need them to be for the purposes of maintaining good health. Before an individual starts eating, try cutting the food in half. Individuals may even feel full before they finish the food. For this reason, they can save the rest of the food for another meal later.

If an individual is overweight then their body knows it and it will probably only ask for a small amount of food. Please do not worry. An individual can eat the next time they are hungry.

If an individual eats beyond full, it may be a very long time before they feel hunger again.

Source: *The Weigh Down Diet* by Gwen Shamblin

Controlling Food Consumption

1. Foods that are high in starch.
These foods give long-lasting energy.
Eat plenty of potatoes, rice, wheat, and other plants.

2. Foods which are high in fiber.
These foods carry food and wastes through the body.
Eat plenty of raw fruits, raw vegetables, wheat, and brown rice, other grains.

3. Foods that are high in cholesterol.
Too much cholesterol can lead to heart disease. This is because cholesterol can clog the arteries.
Cut down on pizza, fried foods, and choose low-fat deserts such as low-fat ice cream.

4. Foods that are high in sodium.
Too much sodium can make the body hold excess fluids. Sodium can also lead to high blood pressure.
Cut down on salty foods and salty snacks. Canned and packaged foods are usually high in sodium.

5. Foods that are high in caffeine.
Too much caffeine can make the heart beat rapidly or irregularly. This can make an individual feel tense.
Cut down on soda and coffee.

6. Foods that are high in sugar.
Sugar provides calories but few nutrients. It contributes to teeth decay.
Cut down on candy, brownies, and cake.

Eating Disorders

An eating disorder is a condition that causes an individual to develop a need to eat food or avoid eating food with the hopes of escaping some type of problem. For example, if Danny is depressed about doing poorly in a Biology class then he will eat 5 pizzas everyday. This shows that Danny may have developed an eating disorder because he is trying to avoid thinking about the fact he did poorly in his class.

In the situation of Danny, he is overeating and this is the most common type of eating disorder among individuals. It can lead to obesity which is being over-weight by at least 20%. Being overweight can cause heart disease, high blood pressure, diabetes, and/or cancer.

Anorexia is an eating disorder in which individuals, usually women, have a fear of becoming fat. For this reason, they put themselves on strict diets. They eat very little food and their bodies do not get the food as well as nutrients they need for healthy lives. Anorexics usually do not feel positive about themselves physically and/or emotionally.

Bulimia is an eating disorder in which people, usually women, will eat food without control (binge). The individuals will then vomit the food for the purpose of getting it out of their stomachs. Getting food out of the stomach is purging. Some individuals living with Bulimia take laxatives to make them go to the bathroom. They want to get rid of the food within their body.

Caffeine and the Body

Caffeine is found in tea, coffee, and some soda drinks. It is a stimulant because it makes the heart beat faster, speeds up the body systems, and makes the individual feel energetic but later brings down their energy level. The effect from drinking soda or coffee that has caffeine can last up to three hours. Coffee without caffeine is called decaffeinated coffee.

Warning about Caffeine

In large quantities, caffeine can harm the stomach lining. It may also put a strain on the hearts of small children. This can lead to death.

Avoid Fried Foods

Fried foods are cooked quickly in fat over a high heat temperature. Individuals should be careful when eating fried foods such as from McDonalds, Burger King, and other restaurants. Fried foods usually have preservatives and chemicals because the restaurants keep the foods in storage for a long period of time. They do not want the foods to get bad quickly because then they have a business loss. The fats and preservatives within the fried foods can lead to heart disease. Heart disease is the most common cause of death in the western world.

The Food Guide Pyramid

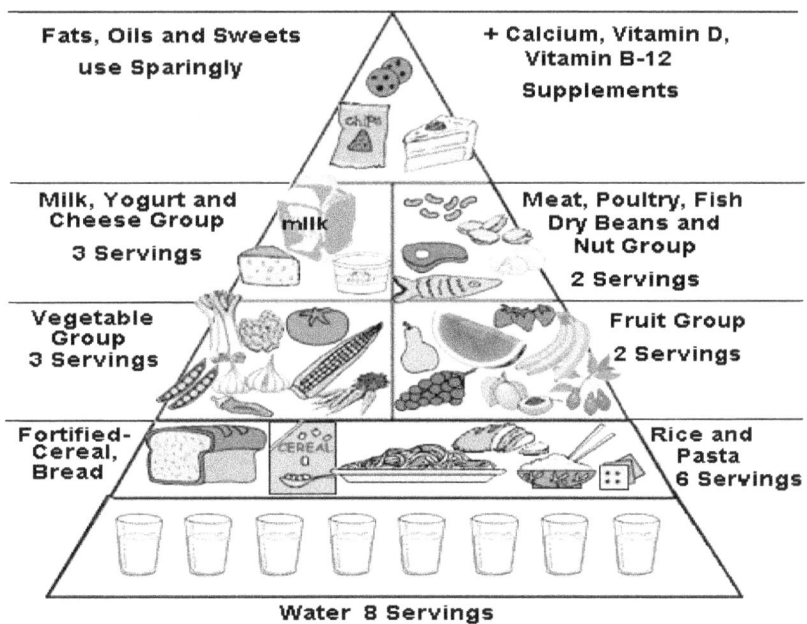

Source: http://www.whale.to/a/food_pyramid.gif

The Food Pyramid was created by the United States Department of Agriculture and United States Department of Health and Human Services as a guide to follow in order to maintain a healthy diet.

Fats, Oils, and Sugar – *recommended to be used sparingly*.
Examples: These are foods such as salad dressings, cream, butter, margarine, sugars, candies, sweet deserts, and soft drinks. This group provides calories to burn for energy.

Milk, Yogurt, and Cheese Group – *recommended 2 to 3 servings a day*.
Examples: One serving is equal to 1 cup milk or yogurt; ½ to 2 ounces cheese. This group provides proteins, minerals, carbohydrates, and vitamins.

Meat, Poultry, Fish, Dry Beans, Eggs, and Nuts Group – *recommended 2 to 3 servings a day*. This group provides proteins, vitamins, and minerals.
Examples: One serving is equal to 2 ½ to 3 ounces of cooked lean meat, poultry, or fish; 1 to 1 ½ cup cooked beans; 1 egg; 4 tablespoons peanut butter.

Vegetable Group – *recommended 3 to 5 servings a day*.
Examples: One serving is equal ½ cup chopped raw or cooked vegetables; 1 cup of leafy raw vegetables. This group provides vitamins, minerals, fiber, and carbohydrates.

Fruit Group – *recommended 2 to 4 servings a day*.

Examples: One serving is equal to 1 piece of fruit or a melon wedge; ¾ cup juice; ½ cup canned fruit; ¼ cup dried fruit. This group provides vitamins, minerals, fiber, and carbohydrates.

Breads, Cereals, Rice, and Pasta Group – *recommended 6 to 11 servings a day*.
Examples: One serving is equal to 1 slice bread; ½ cup cooked rice, pasta, or cereal; 1 ounce cold cereal. This group provides energy, proteins, vitamins, minerals, carbohydrates, and fiber.

Nutrition and Food

Food is made up of nutrients that allow for the body to function, grow, and repair itself.

Fat is a nutrient. The body of an individual can store fat and when necessary, use it later as energy.

Carbohydrates give energy. An example of a source of carbohydrates is white sugar. White sugar is mostly made of a carbohydrate called sucrose.

Protein is used to build the body and almost 20% of the body weight is protein.

Oranges and green vegetables are a source of vitamin C. Vitamin C helps glue body cells together to make firm muscles and smooth skin.

Vitamin A is needed by the body for the production of healthy cells especially those of the digestive system. Vitamin A helps individuals have better vision during the nighttime. This is because vitamin A improves their eyesight.

The human body is about 68% water.

The human body needs small quantities of minerals such as calcium to help make bones and teeth. It also needs iron for healthy blood.

The fat contains twice as much energy as the carbohydrates. During digestion, fats are broken down into fatty acids or glycerol. During prolonged exercise, these substances are converted into energy. Otherwise, the fatty acids and glycerol are stored in the fat cells under the skin and around some organs.

Proteins are broken down into molecules called amino acids. The amino acids are carried within the blood to all the body parts, cells (tissues), and are rearranged into new proteins to form muscles, hair, skin, and blood cells.

Carbohydrates are broken down by the body into glucose and energy is released. If the glucose is not needed then it will be stored in the liver or muscles are glycogen. Extra carbohydrates are converted into fats. Exercise increases the storage of capacity of glycogen so the body stores less fat.

The Six Groups of Nutrients

Nutrients are the parts of the food that the body uses to grow, repair itself, and give energy.

Carbohydrates give the body energy and help in digestion. They include sugars and starches. Carbohydrates can be found in bread, cereal, potatoes, rice, pasta, fruits, and vegetables.

Fats help the human body store energy. They help the body make the chemicals it needs to function, and they help the body use certain vitamins. The layer of fat belonging to the body keeps individuals warm and protects the organs. Fats can be found in butter, margarine, meats, mayonnaise, cheese, and cream foods. Another name individuals use to refer to fats is lipids.

There are 13 different types of vitamins and they all have different functions. Some of the functions include regulating body functions, helping the body use nutrients, and fighting infections. Vitamins can be found in most foods. Fruits and vegetables are especially good sources of vitamins.

Minerals help make muscles and bones strong and healthy. They are found in foods such as meats, milk, fish, and vegetables.

Water helps the body stay at the right temperatures and keeps the digestive system running smoothly. The blood is composed mostly of water. It helps cushion the brain and delicate spinal nerves. Water is found in many foods such as milk, fruits, and juice.

The Effects of Vitamins on the Body

Vitamins that belong to the B group were originally thought to be one substance. Later, it was discovered that there are at least 12 different substances involved with the B group. Some B group vitamins help release energy from food. Others help to make healthy blood and nerves.

Vitamin D is needed for strong bones. The body automatically makes vitamin D when the sunlight is emitting itself on the skin. The bodies of adults usually can make all the vitamin D that is necessary. However, children need extra vitamin D from foods such as eggs, margarine, and oily fish. An example of an oily fish can be sardines. If children do not get enough vitamin D then their bones may not harden properly. As a result, the bones will be more likely to become bent. This condition is called rickets.

Vitamin C is significant for skin, blood, and general body maintenance. It helps healing after an injury because it helps form scar tissue.

Vitamin E protects valuable body chemicals. It makes the blood more efficient in carrying oxygen around the body. Blood carrying oxygen is called oxygenated blood.

Vitamin K helps the blood clot. Without this vitamin, an individual would likely bleed to death when they cut themselves. The human body itself can make a certain amount of vitamin K. Therefore, it is rare to be deficient of the vitamin.

Digestion

It is important that individuals eat normally. However, they should not overeat because such can lead to becoming unhealthy. When an individual eats then they are providing energy to all the parts of the body such as the blood, bones, and brain. Food is the fuel of the body. Individuals should have the proper servings of each food group as recommended by the food guide pyramid.

When an individual eats food then it gets smashed up by the teeth and stomach into a pulp. Juices from the digestive system work on this pulp and break it down into tiny particles called molecules. The molecules are absorbed into the blood and to different parts of the body.

When the food is in the mouth then it gets covered by saliva so it can be made easier for an individual to chew on and digest. The food travels from the mouth to the stomach using the esophagus, which is a long tube in the neck.

In the stomach, the food gets covered by enzymes and it gets broken into even smaller parts so it can go into the small intestine. Any foods or water that the body cannot use or digest goes into the large intestine. The large intestine is sometimes called a colon. The two kidneys in the body pick up any wastes in the small or large intestines and then remove them from the body. Some of the wastes become urine so they can be disposed.

The rate at which chemical processes such as digestion and absorption of the food, take place in the body is called the metabolic rate.

Achieving the Desired Weight

If an individual is underweight then he or she may need to gain weight. They can do so by taking in more calories or burning fewer calories.

If an individual is overweight or obese then he or she needs to lose weight by exercising and eating properly using a food plan or the Food Guide Pyramid.

To maintain a desired weight, an individual should take in the same number of calories that they are able to burn by properly exercising and eating.

To Make Healthy Food Choices

Eat healthful snacks such as yogurt, nuts, raw fruits, raw vegetables, and popcorn.

Follow the Food Guide Pyramid. Eat food from these groups.
-Bread, cereal, rice, and pasta.
-Vegetables.
-Fruits.
-Milk, yogurt, and cheese.
-Meat, poultry, fish, dry beans, eggs, and nuts.

Avoid too much sugar, fats, cholesterol, sodium, and caffeine.

Fitness

Totally Fit
An individual is able to handle physical, mental, emotional, and social day-to-day challenges without feeling exhausted.

When an individual is physically fit then their body is able to handle any type of activity that occurs on a daily basis in their life.

Physical fitness is achieved through 2 types of exercises

1. Aerobic Exercises
Nonstop, repetitive, and vigorous exercises that increase breathing and heart beat rates.

2. Anaerobic Exercises
Involves great bursts of energy in which the muscles work hard to produce energy.

Three Stages of an Exercise Session

Stage 1

Warm-up

A period of mild exercise that gets the body of an individual ready for vigorous activities and exercises.

Stage 2

Workout

Three Workout Factors

1. Frequency.

2. Intensity.

3. Time.

Stage 3

Cool-Down

A period of gentle exercises that gets the body of the individual to stop exercising so the individual can relax.

The Benefits of Exercise

Exercise can help individuals relax and sleep better.

Exercise can help individuals control their weight because it makes the body burn calories at a faster rate.

Exercising makes an individual feel and look good because it gives them more energy and helps firm up the muscles.

Exercise can build muscle strength. Examples of exercises that can achieve this goal include cycling, handball, cross country, skiing, and lifting weights.

Exercise can build heart, lung, and muscle endurance. Examples of exercises that can help achieve this endurance include aerobic exercises, swimming, soccer, and aerobic dancing.

Exercise can promote flexibility. Examples of exercises that can achieve this goal include ballet, tennis, swimming, and volley ball.

Adding Up Your Physical Fitness

Your muscle strength.

+

Your muscle endurance

+

Your flexibility

+

Your heart and lung endurance

+

Your body composition

= The level of physical fitness.

The Organ System

An organ is a group of two or more different tissues (groups of cells) that work together and perform a certain function.

An organ system is a group of organs that work together and perform one or more specific functions within the body. Examples of organ systems are the skeletal system, immune system, cardiovascular system, circulatory system, muscular system, and the lymphatic system.

System
Respiratory

Organs
Lungs, nasal passages (nose and mouth), bronchi, larynx, throat, trachea, diaphragm, and epiglottis.

Functions
-To carry oxygen to the blood.
-To deliver oxygen to the body.
-To remove carbon dioxide from the blood.

System
Nervous

Organs
Spinal cord, brain, and nerves.

Functions
-To send and receive messages.
-To control all body systems.

System
Digestive

Organs
Salivary glands, stomach, liver, teeth, tongue, pancreas, intestines, esophagus, and gallbladder.

Functions

-To break down food an individual eats into a form that the body cells can use as fuel (changes the food into nutrients).

System
Excretory

Organs
Kidneys, bladder.

Functions
-To get rid of wastes.
-To control waster and salt balance of cells.

System
Endocrine

Organs
Glands.

Functions
-To produce hormones to regulate body activities.

System
Skeletal

Organs
Bones, joints, and connecting tissues.

Functions
-To support the body.
-To allow movement.
-To protect organs.

System
Cardiovascular and Circulatory

Organs
Blood, blood vessels, and heart.

Functions

-The transportation system of the body.
-To bring food and oxygen to the cells.
-To take wastes away from the cells.

System
Muscular

Organs
About 600 muscles.

Functions
-To make the body parts move.

Cardiovascular System

The cardiovascular system, sometimes called the circulatory system, is responsible for supplying the body with blood. It pumps the blood from the heart and directs it to the lungs for the purpose of receiving oxygen. After the blood receives the oxygen then it goes back to the heart so it can be distributed throughout the body and its parts such as the brain, kidneys, and other organs. Afterwards, the blood goes back to the heart. This circulation of the blood is repetitive and continuous.

The heart is a muscle, the major organ of the circulatory system. Arteries, capillaries, and veins are the three major types of blood vessels that carry blood throughout the body.

Danger to the Cardiovascular System: Fats

The fatty deposits in the arteries can lead to the blockage of coronary arteries. This eventually means a heart attack. As the fat deposits and increases in the arteries then the heart has to work harder to supply the same amount of blood through the smaller diameter arteries.

Terms to Know

Lungs: Replaces carbon dioxide in the blood with oxygen.

Pulmonary vein: Blood vessel that carries oxygen-rich blood to heart.

Left atrium: Chamber that receives oxygen-rich blood in the heart.

Left ventricle: Chamber that pumps oxygen-rich blood out of the heart.

Aorta: The biggest artery of the human body.

Arteries: Distributes the blood from the heart to smaller blood vessels.

Capillaries: Carries blood to and from body cells.

Veins: Receives low-oxygen blood from small blood vessels.

Right atrium: Chamber that receives low-oxygen blood in the heart.

Right ventricle: Chamber that pumps blood out of the low-oxygen, high carbon-dioxide blood out of the heart back to the lungs.

The Cardiovascular and Circulatory Systems Together

The cardiovascular and circulatory systems are similar because they are responsible for keeping the heart pumping blood every second otherwise the individual could die. The heart valve controls how much blood is released into the body.

The red blood cells are what make the blood red. Blood is blue until it reaches the heart. 80% of the blood is water and for this reason, individuals must drink plenty of water everyday. Usually, if the urine is clean then it suggests the individual is drinking enough water.

Arteries and veins are the blood vessels of the body. However, they are different from each other because arteries are used to circulate blood throughout the human body. In contrast, veins are used to bring blood back to the heart for oxygen as well as nutrients. The blood stream travels through the blood vessels.

The heart is protected by the rib cage that is part of the skeletal system.

In the capillaries, food and oxygen are released to the body cells, and carbon dioxide and other wastes are returned to the bloodstream.

Blood

Blood is a mixture of solids in a large amount of liquid called plasma.

Parts

Plasma is 92% water.

Red blood cells.

White blood cells (lymphocytes).

Platelets help the blood clot.

Blood Vessels

The purpose of them is to circulate the blood throughout the body.

Types
-Arteries.
-Veins.
-Capillaries.

The blood pressure is the pressure of the blood against the walls of the blood vessels.

Blood Types

A

B

AB

O

Blood Pressure

There are two types of blood pressure calculations.

The systolic blood pressure measures the maximum pressure in the blood vessels when the heart beats.

Normal: 139 or less.
Borderline: 140 – 159.
High: 160 or more.

The diastolic blood pressure measures the minimum pressure in the blood vessels between the heart beats.

Normal: 89 or less.
Borderline: 90 – 94.
High: 95 or more.

The cardiac output is the amount of blood pumped by the heart during a certain period of time. It is calculated by doing the Heart Rate times Stroke Volume.

Heart Disease

Heart disease is any condition that lessens the strength or function of the heart or blood vessels. It is the number one killer of adults in the United States.

Body Reactions

1. Heart attack: Blood flow to the heart slows down or stops because the heart muscle tissues die from lack of oxygen.

2. A stroke is a condition in which the blood supply to the brain is disturbed.

A heart attack or stroke can lead to death.

Common Conditions

Atherosclerosis: Fatty substances in the blood deposited on the walls of the arteries.

Arteriosclerosis: The hardening of the arteries and slows the flow of blood.

High blood pressure: When the blood pressure of the individual is higher than normal

Five Risk Factors an Individual Can Control

1. Weight

2. Exercise

3. Diet

4. Stress

5. Tobacco

Respiratory System

The respiratory system provides the body with a continuous supply of oxygen and ridding the body of carbon dioxide.

Parts

Nose and mouth: Where air enters the body.

Throat: Passageway for food and air.

Trachea: Directs air to lungs.

Epiglottis: Tissue that closes over the trachea when an individual swallows food.

Larynx: Contains the vocal cords.

Bronchi: Passages through which air enters the lungs.

Lungs: Where oxygen is put into the blood and carbon dioxide is removed.

Diaphragm: Separates the abdomen from the area around the lungs. It is a muscular wall located below the rib cage.

Diseases

Flu/colds: Communicable disease caused by virus.

Tuberculosis: Bacterial lung infection.

Allergies: Reactions and sensitivity to certain substances.

Pneumonia: Lung infection by bacteria or viruses.

Bronchitis: Swelling of the bronchi due to an infection.

Asthma: Bronchial swelling and blockage.

Emphysema: Alveoli (air sac) destroyed.

Lung cancer: Alveoli (air sac) destroyed and more damaging effects occur with the lungs.

Anatomy of Lungs

Bronchi: Branched part of the lung that holds the alveoli (air sac).

Diaphragm: A muscle below the lungs that draws the air in and pushes it out.

Trachea: Also called the "airway." The tube is connected to the mouth. Without a trachea, it would be impossible for an individual to have the ability to whistle.

Alveoli: Exchanges carbon dioxide for oxygen.

The pulse is a measure of how fast the heart is beating. An individual can take their pulse by feeling their wrist and count how many beats occur within a minute.

Muscular System

The muscular system is the group of tough tissue (cells) that make the body parts move such as the arms, legs, head, and hands.

Muscles work by contracting and extending.

There are 3 major types of muscles, which are smooth muscle, skeletal muscle, and cardiac muscle.

Disorders of the Muscular System

-Pulled or torn muscle.
-Strain.
-Cramp.
-Tendonitis (Sometimes spelled as "tendinitis").
-Muscular dystrophy- Weakens skeletal muscles.

Skeletal and Muscular Systems Together

Muscles are composed of stretchy and elastic cells. Adenosine Triphosphate is ATP. It a chemical found in all living cells and releases energy for cellular reactions. Individuals have over 600 muscles. When a muscle is "working" then this means it is contracting and the muscles are holding the organs in place. The human body has three kinds of muscles. These types are skeletal, smooth, and heart. A muscle can pull but it cannot push. It takes a pair of muscles to bend the human arm back and forth. Muscles that are used to control movements consist of long and thin cells called fibers.

The skeleton is the framework of the body and it is composed of bones. The skeletal system is made up of bones, joints, and connective tissues that help to support, move, and protect the body. The bones in the skull protect the brain. Specifically, the helmet-shaped part of the skull that encloses the brain is the cranium.

There are 206 bones in the body. The bones are joined together at places called joints. The joints are strengthened thanks to tough tissue called ligaments. The joints are lined with cartilage. The ball and socket joint in the body is the shoulder.

A hinge joint in the body is the fingers, toes, elbows, knees, and jaw. The spinal column, sometimes called the backbone, is a series of small bones that enclose and protect the spinal cord. The 33 small ring-shaped bones that make up the spinal column are called vertebrae. The 12 pairs of curved bones attached to the spinal column are the ribs. Several pairs of ribs are joined by connective tissue to the sternum, or breastbone. The bowl-shaped bone at the hips is called the pelvis.

The hollow part of each bone contains marrow. The red marrow makes blood cells such as the white blood cells. The white blood cells are considered lymphocytes that are part of the immune system. They help defend the body against diseases and infections such as the common cold.

Ossification is the process of forming bones. Cartilage is a tough, flexible connective tissue, which is found wherever two or more bones come together.

The Three Parts of the Skeletal System

1. Bones have 5 jobs. They help the individual with movement, support, protection, blood cell formation, and storage.

2. Joints come in 4 types, which are the pivot, ball-and-socket, hinge, and gliding.

3. Connectors, which come in 3 types of tissues: cartilage, ligaments, and tendons.

Diseases of the Skeletal System

1. The swelling of a joint because of twisted ligaments: Sprain.

2. A curvature of the spine: Scoliosis.

3. A break or crack in a bone as a result of an accident: Fracture.

4. Swollen and stiff joints, usually afflicting older people: Arthritis.

5. A bone pushed out of the joint: Dislocation.

6. Brittle, porous bones often caused by lack of calcium: Osteoporosis.

Foot Problems

Type
Callus.

Location
Heel or back of foot.

Description
Hard, thickened skin, caused by foot rubbing against the shoe.

Type
Corn.

Location
Toe.

Description
Overgrowth of skin from toe rubbing against shoe.

Type
Blister.

Location
Skin.

Description
Fluid-filled pouch formed by ill-fitting shoes.

Type
Bunion.

Location
First joint of big toe.

Description
Inflammation caused by tight shoes.

Type
Athlete's foot.

Location
Warm, damp areas of foot.

Description
Redness and itching caused by fungi.

Type
Fallen arches.

Location
Bottom of feet.

Description
Flatness caused by weakening of muscles and tissues.

Building Bones and Teeth

Bones consist of protein and water filled in with calcium phosphate. This is made up of 2 materials, which are calcium and a little phosphorus. Calcium is found mainly in milk, cheese, cereals, and vegetables. Vitamin D is used to help create and strengthen bones.

Teeth are mostly made of calcium but individuals also need another mineral called fluoride. Fluoride helps with the enamel coating and can help prevent tooth decay. Fluoride is found in the water supply in some locations.

Central Nervous System and Peripheral Nervous System

Central Nervous System (CNS)

Serves as the main control center of the human body.

Parts of the CNS

-Spinal cord: Relays messages.
-Brain: Controls actions, emotions, thoughts, and memories.

Peripheral Nervous System (PNS)

Carry messages to and from the central nervous system.

Parts of the PNS

-Somatic system: Deals with actions an individual controls.
-Autonomic system: Deals with actions an individual cannot control.

Nervous System and Associated Disorders

The nervous system is the brain and spinal cord working together to send messages throughout the body using nerve cells. The messages tell the body how to function. For example, in simplest terms, if an individual wants to walk then their brain will send a message for the legs to walk and the muscles will also comply with this message. The message will travel using the spinal cord and nerve cells. Problems with the nervous system can cause an individual to possibly become disabled or one of their body parts could become dysfunctional in some aspect.

Disorder
Epilepsy

Cause
Brain disorder in which there are irregular electrical discharges

Description
It causes uncontrollable muscle activity and may cause the individual to become unconscious

Treatment
Controlled by medication prescribed by a doctor

Disorder
Polio

Cause
By a virus

Description
It can result in a person developing paralysis, which is the inability to use muscles

Treatment
Vaccination

Disorder
Cerebral palsy

Cause

Damage or injury to the cerebrum

Description
Symptoms vary but usually there is a lack of muscle control particularly with the limbs

Treatment
Unfortunately, there is no cure but therapy can help victims try and live normal lives

Disorder
Multiple Sclerosis

Cause
Damage or injury to the protective outer coating of some of the nerve cells

Description
Weakness with the muscles, eyesight, and slow speech as well as the inability to move

Treatment
There is no cure but medication and therapy can help in the early stages of the disorder

Disorder
Rabies

Cause
A virus causes the disorder and the virus enters the body of the individual when the individual is bitten by an infected animal

Description
It can cause an individual to have unusual behavior, their body may uncontrollably shake, they may struggle to move, and it may lead to death

Treatment
Series of shots, medications, and individuals need to avoid possibly infected animals

Any injury to the nervous system or disorder is very serious because it may lead to the individual becoming paralyzed in some aspect. This means they will lose the ability to move one or more of the parts belonging to their body. For example, an individual who loses the ability to walk due to paralysis will have to use a wheelchair their entire life.

Immune System

A disease is an unhealthy condition of the body or mind that causes the body not to function properly. The individual may struggle to live their everyday normal life living with a disease.

The First Line of Defense

The barriers such as the skin are the first defense against disease.

Skin and mucous membranes in the nose, mouth, and throat keep the germs out. The skin is considered to be the physical barrier. The mucous membranes are considered the digestive, respiratory, and genitourinary barriers.

Saliva tears and gastric juices wash germs away or attack them with chemicals.

The most common disease causing organisms are virus, bacteria, and fungi.

Secretions of skin and mucous membranes

-Oil and sweat glands make skin pH 3-5.
-Washing acting of saliva, tears, and mucous.
-Antimicrobial protein such as the lysozome. This is found in tears, saliva, and the mucous digests bacterial cell walls.
-Mucus traps microbes and swept out by the cilia. The cilia are located in the trachea.
-Most microbes are destroyed by the acid of the stomach.

The Second Line of Defense

Phagocytic white blood cell: Ingests microbes.

1. Neutrophiles: 60 to 70% of white blood cells (leukocytes).
-By chemotaxis = Movement toward the source of chemical attractant.
-They self-destruct as they destroy microbes.

2. Monocytes: 5% of white blood cells
-Most effective.
-Develops into macrophages ("big eaters").
-Extends pseudopods that attach to polysacs on microbe surface and eat microbe, then destroyed by enzymes. Some microbes have outer capsules to which macs cannot

attack. For example, *Mycobacterium tuberculosis* is resistant to the Lysosome destruction and can reproduce in mac.
-Macs in lung, connective tissue, brain, tissue, kidney, liver, lymph nodes, and spleen.

3. Eosinophils: 1.5% of white blood cells
-Against larger parasites (blood flukes – Schistosoma).
-Secrete enzymes that destroy microbe.
-Limited phagocytosis.

NK Cells (Natural Killer)
-Destroy the virus-infected body cells and cancerous cells.
-Not phagocytic.
-Lyse body cell membrane.

Inflammatory Response
-Initiated by chemical signals.
-Histamine produced by basophils and mast cells. This begins dilation and increases the permeability of capillaries.
-Prostaglandins from white blood cells and damaged cells. This increases blood flow.

Increased the flowage of blood and permeability
-Deliver clotting elements such as the blood clot repairs and blocks spread of microbes.
-Increases phagocytes from blood. This is controlled by the chemokines.
-Neutrophils are first then monocytes, which transform in to macs. The macs eat the damaged cells, microbes, and the remains of neutrophiles.

Pus is dead phags, fluid, and protein from caps. This is absorbed by the body after a few days.

Localized Inflammation versus Systemic Inflammation

-Systemic response equals whole body (not local area).
-Fever triggered by:
1. Microbe toxins.
2. Pyrogens (chemicals released by white blood cells). The increased temperature kills the microbes and increases enzyme activity for the repair of tissues.

Antimicrobial Proteins
1. This is a complement system that equals 20 serum proteins that lyse microbes.
2. Interferons
-Released by the cells infected by the virus.
-Diffuse to non-virus-infected cells to inhibit viral reproduction.
-This helps prevent the spreading of influenza or the common cold.
-Research is used to produce interferons to fight cancer and viruses.

The Third Line of Defense

Lymphocytes are a type of white blood cell.
-Provide the diversity and specificity of the immune system.

There are 2 types.
1. B cells.
2. T cells.

Found in blood, lymph, concentrated in spleen, and lymph nodes.

Specific: Recognize and respond to specific microbes and foreign molecules.

Antigen: "Antibody-generator" which means the microbe or foreign molecule that elicits certain response by lymphocytes such as bacteria, fungi, virus, protozoa, parasitic worms, pollen, transplanted cells, cancerous cells, and sperm in females.

Antibody: Specific protein secreted by activated B cells in response to a specific antigen.

Antigen Receptors: Proteins on the lymphocyte cell membrane that recognizes specific antigen. There are about 100,000 identical receptors on each cell. The genetic information forms diversity of lymphocytes to respond to millions of different antigens. This can include antigens that may not have yet been developed.

1. On the B cells = "Membrane antibodies or immunoglobulins."
2. On the T cells = "T cell receptors."

Antigens interact with specific lymphocytes, inducing immune responses and immunological memory.

Clonal selection: Antigen "selects" a specific lymphocyte to bind is based on the shape of the antigen and shape of the receptor. Afterwards, the antigen activates the lymphocyte to reproduce (proliferate), producing thousands of "clones" (identical copies) to help get rid of the antigen.

Two types of clones are produced:

1. Effector cells: Short-lived cells that fight the same antigen.

In B cells, the effector cells are called the "plasma cells." These cells produce antibodies specific for antigens. In T cells, the effector cells are called the "effector T cells" and they do not produce antibodies.

2. Memory cells: Long-lived cells that respond quickly upon another exposure to specific antigen.

Primary Immune Response
Clonal selection when the first is exposed to the antigen. The response time is usually ten to seventeen days. This is the time during which the person may become ill.

Secondary immune response is the response upon subsequent exposure to the same antigen. The response time is usually about two to seven days. There is greater magnitude because more antibodies are produced. This lasts longer and explains why an individual does not usually get chickenpox a second time.

Development of Lymphocyte
Pluripotent stem cells in red bone marrow or fetal liver. These cells transform into lymphocytes and later into B or T cells. Pluripotent means the cell has the ability to differentiate into any type of blood cell.

B cells mature within the bone marrow. This was first discovered in bursa of Fabricius in birds. In contrast, the T cells mature in the thymus gland.

Self-tolerance: The capacity of the immune system to distinguish self from nonself. Programmed cell death may happen if the lymphocyte has receptors specific for "self" molecules or the lymphocyte made nonfunctional.

Autoimmune disease is the failure of self-tolerance. Examples can include multiple sclerosis (MS), lupus, rheumatoid arthritis, and insulin-dependent diabetes mellitus.

Cell Surface Makers on T Cells

Major histocompatibility complex (MHC): Cell surface glycoproteins on body cells that mark cells as "self" and present the antigen to a T cell. This is also known as human leukocyte antigens (HLA).

There are 2 main classes of MHC molecules:

1. Class 1 MHC: On all nucleated cells (most cells in body).

2. Class II MHC: On macrophages, B cells, activated T cells, and inferior thymus cells.

Except identical twins, no two people have exactly the same set of MHC (hundreds of possible alleles for gene) = Biochemical fingerprint. This was discovered when studying tissue grafts. Histo means "tissue."

Antigen Presentation
MHC cradles fragment of antigen and presents it to the T cell.

2 Main Types of T Cells

1. Cytotoxic T cell: Bind to Class 1 MHC.

2. Helper T cell: Bind to Class 2 MHC.

Any MHC can present a variety of antigen fragments. MHC-antigen complex is recognized by the specific antigen receptors on T cells. T cells maturing in the thymus differentiate into cytotoxic and helper T cells by their interactions with the thymus cells. The thymus cells have both Class 1 and Class 2 MHC.

General Reactions

Special blood cells may surround and destroy the germs. These cells may initiate the body to release chemicals that will destroy any viruses. The body may raise the temperature with a fever for the purpose of killing the remaining germs. They cannot survive in a hot environment.

After the first line of defense, the immune system is the next defense against diseases. The Immune system Is a group of cells and organs that fight specific germs.

Lymphocytes are the white blood cells of the immune system that fight germs. They are the T and B cells. The T cells detect the germs and call upon the B cells that then create antibodies for the specific germs.

The T cells detect germs because they recognize the antigens, the unique chemicals on the surface of a germ.

Due to the fact that the B cells made antibodies for the specific germs, if they were to enter the body again then they would be destroyed immediately. This is because the body now has immunity to them. Immunity is considered resistance to the infection.

Defense of the Human Body

- The skin of the human body weighs 6 pounds.

- The lymph nodes contain billions of white blood cells (lymphocytes). They multiply rapidly within the body when they fight infections and/or germs.

- The spleen is behind the stomach on the left side. It makes and stores various types of white blood cells, especially the phagocytes that eliminate the germs.

- The tonsils are patches of lymph tissue at the upper rear part of the throat. Tonsils help to destroy foreign substances that are breathed in or swallowed by an individual.

- The thymus gland in the front of the chest is large during childhood. However, it shrinks away during adulthood. It produces the T cells, which are the white blood cell lymphocytes.

Endocrine System

The endocrine system helps individuals undergo puberty. The system helps the individual physically and mentally mature into an adult. This system also regulates the glands that secrete the chemicals needed for development.

Glands

Pituitary gland (Master gland): Controls other glands.

Thyroid: Regulates calcium and phosphorus in the body.

Pancreas: Controls blood sugar levels.

Ovaries: Reproduction in females.

Testes: Reproduction in males.

Adrenal: Controls response to emergencies.

Parathyroid: Controls how the body uses food for fuel.

Excretory System

The excretory system is responsible for getting rid of wastes from the body.

Functions

Excretes water: Kidneys, lungs, and skin.

Excretes carbon dioxide: Lungs.

Excretes urea: Kidneys.

Excretes salt: Kidneys and skin.

Helps maintain body temperature: Lungs.

Produces urine: Kidneys.

Brings oxygen to blood: Lungs.

Reproductive System

Organs involved in the production of offspring, which is a baby, are part of the reproductive system.

Organs

Males

Ejaculation: Process by which sperm cells leave the body.

Fertilization: Union of an egg and sperm.

Ovulation: Process in which an egg cell is released from an ovary.

Penis: Male organ for urination and reproduction.

Semen: Liquid containing sperm cells.

Uterus: Pear-shaped organ in which the fertilized egg develops into a baby.

Females

Menstruation takes place when the lining of the uterus, sometimes called the womb, breaks down and passes out of the body as blood. When this happens then the woman has had a period. The lining of the uterus is the blood that is meant to help with the creation of a baby in the event the woman becomes pregnant. The time from 1 menstruation to the next is called the menstrual cycle.

A gynecologist is a doctor who specializes in treating the female reproductive system. A common problem of the female reproductive system is vaginitis, which is inflammation. The woman will feel pain and itching on their genitals. Vaginitis may sometimes be a result of infection.

The glands of the male that produce sperm are called the testes, sometimes called the testicles. Sperm produced in the testes are stored in the epididymis. A sperm is a male reproductive cell.

Males and females need to be careful when lifting heavy objects. This is because if they often lift them incorrectly then they may develop an inguinal hernia.

Female Reproductive System

The time during which a young female individual begins to mature and release eggs is puberty. The female sex hormones are oestrogen and progesterone. These hormones help develop the secondary sexual characteristics of a female. One characteristic is the development of wider hips.

The stage at which an older female individual stops having periods due to the fact their body is no longer releasing eggs is menopause.

The female gamete is the ovum and egg. The female gonad is the ovary. The oviduct is also called the fallopian tube. In the fallopian tube is where conception or fertilization occurs within a female individual. The stage at which an ovum (egg) is released from the ovary is called ovulation.

The womb is sometimes called the uterus. The average gestation period of an individual is 40 weeks. This is when the woman carries the baby in the womb.

Days 1 to 5 of the menstrual cycle are the stages of menstruation. During pregnancy, a woman does not have periods.

Menstruation

1. The uterus has the lining, which is the blood.

2. The lining gets thicker.

3. The lining flows out of the uterus. This is when the woman has the period.

4. The menstrual cycle starts again.

Ovulation: The releasing of an egg from the ovary

1. The ovum is the egg. It bursts from the ovary.

2. Finger-like projections pull the egg into the fallopian tube.

3. The egg travels through the fallopian tube on its way into the uterus.

4. The egg travels to the uterus and attaches itself to the lining where it is shed unless it has been fertilized.

Female Reproductive Anatomy

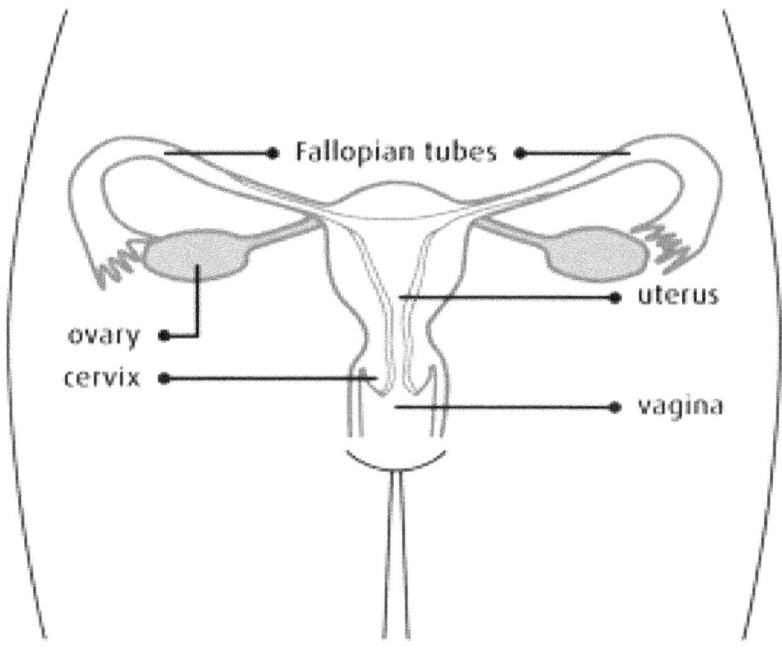

Source: http://www.cancer.ca/Canada-wide/About%20cancer/Types%20of%20cancer/~/media/CCS/Canada%20wide/Images%20list/English%20Images/Graphics/Uterine-Cervical-Ovarian%20-%20UYD%20-%20Diagram%20-%20English%202007_1494300965.ashx

Cervix: Neck-like, narrow end of uterus which open into the vagina. It stretches to allow a baby to be born.

Vagina: Passage that leads from uterus to external genital organs.

Uterus (womb): Pear-shaped female reproductive organ in which the fetus grows and develops until birth.

Fallopian tubes: There are 2 fallopian tubes. Through 1 of the tubes, an egg is released from an ovary every month and travels on its way to the uterus.

Ovary: Female organ in which egg cells and sex hormones are produced.

Male Reproductive Anatomy

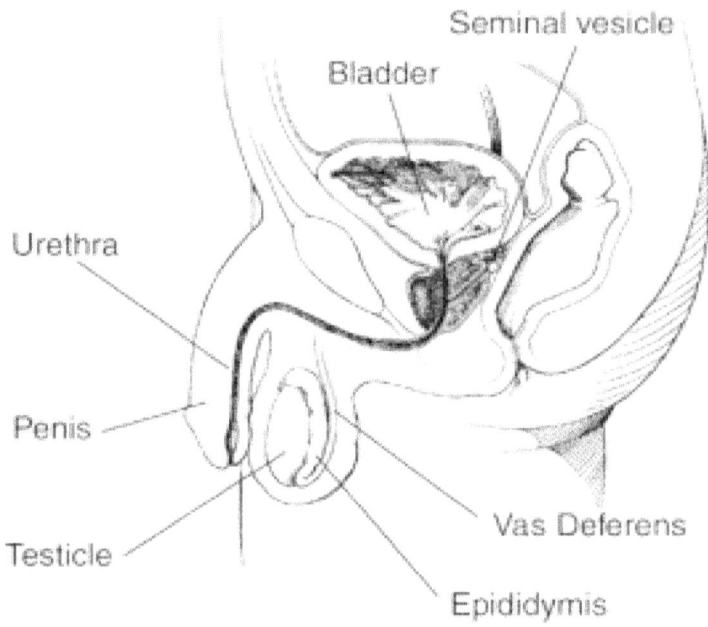

Source: http://www.uroncology.com/images/52196-1.gif

Penis: The male sex organ; also, the male urinary organ.

Urethra: The duct through which urine is discharged. In males, this is the duct through which semen is discharged. If the urethra is blocked or any problems occur with it then a male could have problems having children.

Scrotum: The external pouch that contains the testicles.

Testicle: The gland that produces sperm.

Vas deferens: The two tubes that allow sperm to pass from the testicles.

Reproduction Terms to Know

Puberty: The physical developmental stage when an individual beings to develop certain traits of their gender. Signs of puberty include emotional swings, menstrual periods and erections, and oil and sweat glands become more active.

Eggs: The fallopian tubes contain the eggs. They are the reproductive cells of the female.

Sperm: They are the reproductive cells of the male and have tails to move within semen.

Semen: White fluid from the penis containing the sperm cells. It is released during sexual intercourse. The semen nourishes them. During puberty, the male will sometimes release semen.

Ovulation: The stage in which an egg is released from the ovary.

Menstrual period (sometimes called "menstruation" or a "period"): The monthly bleeding that occurs with the female when the blood and other matter from the womb are released.

Erection: The stage in which the penis becomes hard because it fills with blood during sexual intercourse.

Fertilization (sometimes called "conception"): The joining of an egg and sperm.

Umbilical cord: The cord that is attached to the fetus and placenta, through which the fetus receives oxygen, nutrients, and food.

Placenta: The protective coating inside the uterus that supplies the fetus with nutrients and oxygen.

Labor: The muscle contractions, or pains, a woman feels before and during birth.

Abstinence: Not having sexual intercourse.

Sexual harassment: When an individual inappropriately harasses another individual and it is sexual in some aspect. Examples can include touching the individual or making advances towards them. An example of a sexual advance can be kissing an individual.

Reproduction: Produce offspring.

Embryo: A fertilized egg.
Maturity: Fully developed emotionally and physically individual.

Biological Development Stages of a Baby

1. Fertilization

A. A protective coating forms around the egg cell.

B. The fertilized cell attaches itself to the wall of the uterus.

C. A sperm cell joins with an egg cell.

D. The placenta begins to provide nourishment to the developing baby.

2. Development before Birth

A. The heart begins to beat.

B. The arms and legs can move freely.

C. The heartbeat can be heard.

D. Body organs have developed enough to work on their own.

3. Birth Process

A. Contraception begins.

B. The contractions become stronger.

C. The cervix opens to a width of about 4 inches.

D. Contractions push the placenta out of the body belonging to the mother.

E. The baby is born. ☺

Pregnancy Myths and Facts

1. A fetus is protected from the drug usage of the mother thanks to the placenta.
False. Drugs negatively affect the development of the fetus through the abnormalities that occur with the blood and cells of the mother.

2. Physical maturity and emotional maturity develop at different rates.
True. For this reason, even though an individual may be physically ready for sexual intercourse, it does not mean they are emotionally ready for it.

3. Abstinence is a physically and emotionally healthy choice.
True. Abstinence is a decision that has no cons but only pros.

Danger behind Pregnancy before Marriage

**Note: This chapter is <u>not</u> meant to insult or underestimate women in any aspect and the chapter is not influenced by religious beliefs.

Individuals are discouraged from having sexual intercourse before marriage especially if they are a teenager or a younger individual. This is because it is possible for the male partner to impregnate the female partner and later leave her during the pregnancy. The male partner may be immature or not desire to handle the responsibilities of raising a child.

As a result, it is likely that the female individual will have to take care of the child without any help or support especially if she has no parents or other family members. It will be extremely difficult for the female individual to carry a child, work a job, and take care of themselves. Getting a job may be a major challenge itself because women are more likely to drop out of school when they become pregnant. This is because some employers require a high school diploma or college degree.

Without marriage, the woman cannot get alimony from the male individual who got her pregnant. She may be able to get child support. However, from my mother's personal experiences, child support is not always enough money to raise a child. The male individual may refuse to pay child support. For this reason, the woman will have to take the male individual to court and hire an attorney. Doing so will likely cost the female individual thousands of dollars and there is no guarantee that she will win the case.

The female individual may feel a great deal of stress during the pregnancy. This will raise the likelihood of the woman having a miscarriage or a premature birth. The can negatively affect the health of the woman. In some cases, she can lose her life.

Some individuals think it is okay to have sexual intercourse before marriage because the woman is safe from becoming pregnant. They think contraception methods will prevent pregnancy. No contraception method is 100% effective against protecting the woman from pregnancy or contracting a sexually transmitted disease. To a certain extent, if one or both of the partners are so worried about the contraception method not working then it may suggest that they are not ready to raise a child.

After the pregnancy, a single mother raising a child is still no easy task. I have witnessed many female students at my community college trying to earn degrees so they can provide a better future for their children. For this reason, I encourage all male individuals who impregnate female individuals to help support their children. There is no excuse for individuals not taking care of their kids.

Teenager Help Hotlines

Teen Hotline: (407) 841-7413.

Crisis Hotline: (407) 425-2624.

Central Florida Helpline: (407) 740-7477.

Sexually Transmitted Diseases (STDs)

Human Immunodeficiency Virus (HIV)

-HIV causes AIDS (Acquired Immune Deficiency Syndrome).

-Virus attacks the immune system. It damages and infects the white blood cells.

-Virus spreads through contact with infected semen, blood, or fluids from the vagina. An infected mother can pass on the virus to her children.

-No cure.

-Symptoms include a rash, sore throat, fever, and tiredness (fatigue).

-People with AIDS cannot fight off diseases that healthy people can fight off easily.

-Abstinence and not sharing needles can prevent HIV.

Syphilis

-Attacks many parts of the body.

-Early symptoms include a reddish, painless sore at the place where the disease entered the body.

-Fatal without treatment.

-Cured with antibodies.

Chlamydia

-Most common sexually transmitted disease in the United States.

-Symptoms include pain and unusual liquid released from the penis or vagina.

-Cured with antibiotics.

-Attacks reproductive organs.

Genital Herpes

-Caused by herpes simplex type II virus.

-Symptoms include a fever and painful, itchy sores where the disease enters the body.

-No cure.

Gonorrhea

-Bacteria that causes it usually to live in warm and moist areas of the body.

-Infection.

-Symptoms include an inside burning feeling during urination.

-Cured with antibodies.

-Unusual liquid coming from the penis or vagina.

HIV Review

Macrophages are white blood cells. Lymphocytes are also white blood cells.

When a body has HIV then it often gets rare illnesses.

Pneumocystic carinii is a rare type of pneumonia, which is the inflammation of the lungs.

Human immunodeficiency virus is the microorganism that causes AIDS.

There is no cure for HIV. A victim of HIV is infected for life.

When an individual is infected, HIV is found in all body fluids.

The best way to avoid HIV is to avoid sexual and blood-to-blood contact with individuals living with HIV.

Facts and Myths about AIDS and HIV

1. HIV weakens the immune system of the body.
-Fact.

2. Injecting drugs with injected needles can spread HIV.
-Fact.

3. Unborn babies can get HIV from their mothers.
-Fact.

4. There is nothing people can do to avoid getting AIDS.
-Myth.
*Individuals can avoid sexual contact with individuals who have HIV or AIDS and should only have sexual intercourse with their committed spouse. Individuals should not touch the bloody wounds or cuts of other individuals.

5. There is no cure for AIDS.
-Fact.

6. People can catch HIV from infected mosquitoes.
-Myth.
*There has never been a case in which an individual became infected with HIV or AIDS due to a mosquito bite.

7. One way to get HIV is to give blood.
-Myth.
*Reputable hospitals and medical centers use safe, secure, clean, and proper equipment to collect blood from donors. They are never allowed to use dirty needles or equipment to collect blood.

8. Carriers can spread HIV even though they show no signs of the virus themselves.
-Fact.

9. There is no way to determine if an individual has AIDS or HIV.
-Myth.
*Individuals can have a blood check done on them. Before having sexual contact with someone, the individual should ask for a medical or blood test report. It should raise concerns if an individual often gets ill. They may have HIV and the individual should avoid sexual contact with them until they know their potential partner does not have the virus.

10. Being infected with HIV makes it possible for other pathogens to attack the body.
-Fact.

11. Shaking hands with an AIDS patient can spread the disease.
-Myth.
*Shaking hands is not blood-to-blood contact and there has never been a case in which an individual became infected with AIDS due to shaking hands. However, if an individual is shaking hands with another individual who has blood on their hands then it may spread the virus.

12. One way to get AIDS is to touch something an AIDS infected individual has touched.
-Myth.
*HIV or AIDS cannot survive on objects outside of a human.

13. Saying no to sexual relations is a good way to avoid getting infected with HIV.
-Fact.

14. The blood used for transfusions during operations today has been tested and probably does not contain HIV.
-Fact.

Genomes are the Salvation from HIV

Genomes are the sets of chromosomes that organisms inherit from their parents. The chromosomes contain genes, which have the information that will determine the biological development of the organism such as their physical aspects including skin color, hair color, and gender. Genomes help determine the structures and functions of inner body organs and cells. Research and studies are showing that if scientists can make certain manipulations with genomes then they may be able to prevent organisms from being infected by the Human Immunodeficiency Virus, which is abbreviated as HIV. HIV is a deadly virus that humans can become infected with through sexual or blood contact with a person that already has HIV. "There are 2 types HIV, which are HIV-1 and HIV-2 and some studies show the HIV-1 can develop into HIV-2," which is usually more lethal. For this reason, people living with HIV are encouraged to live the healthiest lives possible especially for the purpose of trying to keep the symptoms of HIV from growing out of control. When HIV enters the body, it detects the helper T cells of the immune system by recognizing the proteins on the surface of the cells called CD4 receptors. A protein is a substance that has linked and is part of the structure of all living cells. HIV uses the CD4 receptors to go into the T cells and changes the function of the T cells, which is normally to protect the body from viruses, infections, and cancers. This is because the T cells are considered white blood cell lymphocytes. Additionally, the T cells are known as thymus cells because they are developed by an organ of the immune system called a "thymus that is located at the neck base." With HIV, the T cells are now used to make more HIV cells and in this sense, HIV reproduces itself and spreads to cells throughout the body. The only way HIV can survive in the body is by reproducing more of itself. Therefore, the T cells have been destroyed, the immunity is weakened in the body, and as the HIV cells spread, the numbers of white blood cells decrease within the body. In fact, a low number of white blood cells can indicate to medical physicians if an individual has HIV. An individual living with HIV usually tends to get ill more often than other individuals living without HIV. A low number of white blood cells can result in the person developing AIDS. AIDS is a disease of the immune system that causes individuals to lose the ability to fight infections. As a result, these individuals pass away from secondary causes such as a stroke.

There is much history connected to HIV. This is because there are many myths and theories as to how it was born. Some people used to think only individuals who were lesbian or homosexual were prone to be infected with the disease due to sexual contact with the same gender whereas other people thought HIV was a punishment given by God to individuals who committed wrong doings. These myths were later proven wrong. HIV was thought by some individuals to be created by some individual but as of now, most research is suggesting HIV evolved from the Simian Immunodeficiency Virus, which can be abbreviated as SIV. SIV is a virus found in primates and has a similar cellular structure compared to HIV. Similar to how HIV causes individuals to be susceptible to many illnesses, SIV causes primates to be susceptible to many illnesses. A personal inference has been made that the individuals living in Cameroon were hunting for chimpanzees to eat as food. They may have been the first individuals to eat the chimpanzees that were living with SIV. When SIV entered their human bodies, its cellular structure changed to adapt to the biological environment of a human. SIV then transformed into HIV. Cameroon is a country located in West Africa. Tests were done with the feces of the chimpanzees living there and SIV was found within the chimpanzees. Cameroon has the greatest population of chimpanzees living with SIV than any other country. Another personal inference is that a primate living with SIV may have attacked a human and the blood contact caused SIV to transfer into the human. Old medical records show some individuals had conditions and symptoms that doctors could not understand. It is likely they were the first individuals that were infected with HIV. Currently, scientists are trying to determine how primates became infected with SIV. This is because if primates were to be cured of SIV then this may lead to a treatment for HIV.

One way scientists may be able to prevent and possibly treat HIV is through gene therapy. Gene therapy is the treatment of diseases by replacing damaged or missing genes with healthy genes. The healthy genes are scientifically created in a laboratory. A study conducted by Dr. Robin Kimmel of Stanford University shows in order for HIV to enter the immune system cells, another protein called "CCR5 along with CD4 are needed." CD4 and CCR5 work together to allow for HIV to enter the cells. The people who are immune towards HIV infections have a mutation with the CCR5 gene known as CCR5-delta32. The CCR5-delta32 mutation creates a smaller protein that is not on the surface of the immune system cells anymore. As a result, HIV cannot detect the immune system cells to infect because they do not have the CCR5 receptors. For this reason, individuals with multiple copies of the CCR5-delta32 gene due to inheritance from parents are strongly immune to HIV. Scientists need to use gene therapy and structure the genes of humans so that their T cells develop the CCR5-delta32 gene mutation. This could be a possible goal of the Human Genome Project. The only ethical problem is that most likely, such therapy would need to be tested on primates living with SIV for the purpose of observing if their disease is treated. Gene therapy can be lethal in the beginning and may cause more harm than good. It could potentially increase the symptoms of the disease and this could result in the death of the primates. As a personal opinion, this is a risk that will need to be taken because HIV is becoming a plague to society. As support, statistics show about "two to two point four million people in the United States have passed away due to HIV." Thankfully, gene therapy has been done on mice and made them immune towards the HIV infection but the problem rises that mice and humans are two different species. The immune systems of the mice developed antibodies called "antibodies called b12 and VRC01." The immunity of the mice suggests that a treatment for HIV will be found soon.

Works Cited

Kimmel, R.. Can genes stop HIV? Stanford School of Medicine, 2004.
Web. 1 Dec 2011. <http://www.thetech.org/genetics/news.php?id=13>.

"Gene Therapy Can Protect against HIV : Nature News & Comment." Nature Publishing
Group : Science Journals, Jobs, and Information. Web. 06 Dec. 2011.
http://www.nature.com/news/gene-therapy-can-protect-against-hiv-1.9516.

Balazs, A. B. et al. Nature advance online publication
http://dx.doi.org/10.1038/nature10660 (2011).
Johnson, P. R. et al. Nature Med. 15, 901-906 (2009).

Common Communicable Diseases

A communicable disease is an illness that an infected person will give to another individual through some means of contact such as touching or kissing. Communicable diseases can be caused by viruses. Individuals are not born with communicable diseases. For example, cancer is not a communicable disease but a non-communicable disease. This is because it is impossible for an individual living with cancer to give another individual cancer even if they had any type of contact. Individuals are sometimes born with non-communicable diseases especially if it runs in their family.

Disease
Common Cold
*Most common upper respiratory infection.

Symptoms
-Mild fever.
-Runny nose.
-Itchy eyes.
-Sneezing.
-Coughing.
-Sore throat.
-Headaches.

Cause
-100 different viruses and germs.

Treatment
-Rest.
-Liquids.
-Over-the-counter (OTC) medications.
-Do not share eating utensils.
-Exercise.
-Balanced diet.
-Avoid smoking.
-Get 8 hours of sleep.

Disease
Mononucleosis
*It is sometimes called the "kissing disease" because individuals can get it through kissing. It is a viral infection and it will cause the swelling of the lymph nodes in the neck and throat.

Symptoms
-Tiredness (fatigue).
-Loss of appetite.
-Fever.
-Sore throat.

Cause
-Direct and indirect contact.

Treatment
-Pain relievers (limited amount).
-Rest.
-Liquids.

Disease
Hepatitis A

Symptoms
-Yellowing of the skin and the eyes may become whiter.

Cause
-Virus.

Treatment
-No cure.
-Rest.
-Gamma globulin (antibody in the bloodstream that fights infection).

Disease
Hepatitis B

Symptoms
-Yellowing of the skin and the eyes may become whiter.

Cause
-Virus

Treatment
-No cure.
-Rest.
-Vaccine.

-Balanced diet.

*An individual can find out if they have hepatitis by agreeing to do a blood test.

Disease
Influenza
*It is usually called "the flu" and it is a respiratory infection.

Symptoms
-Tiredness (fatigue).
-Chills.
-Headaches.
-Body aches.
-Respiratory problems.
-Fever.

Cause
-Direct and indirect contact.
-Sneezing.
-Coughing.

Treatment
-Yearly vaccines may help prevent the illness.
-Rest.
-Balanced diet.
-Medicine.

Disease
Tuberculosis

Symptoms
-Usually affects the lungs.
-Spread by coughing or sneezing.
-Symptoms include fever, fatigue, weight loss, coughing, and blood loss.

Cause
-Bacteria.

Treatment
-Long-term use of antibodies.

Means through how Germs Spread
-Direct contact.
-Indirect contact.
-Contact with animals.
-Sexual contact.
-Other contacts.

Avoid Germs!
-Bacteria.
-Viruses.
-Rickettsias.
-Fungi.
-Protozoa.

Noncommunicable Diseases and their Causes

Noncommunicable diseases cannot be spread by person to person such as how the common cold spreads among people. They are caused by heredity (acquired genetic traits from parents), unhealthy lifestyles or habits (usage of drugs or unhealthy eating), and the hazards in the environment, water, or buildings.

4 Noncommunicable Diseases

Heart Disease

The types include arteriosclerosis, atherosclerosis, stroke, and high blood pressure (hypertension). They are usually caused by an excessive build up of fat within the arteries. Medication, surgery, and changes in the lifestyle can treat heart disease.

Cancer

It is caused by abnormal cells growing out of control. It may start as a mass of abnormal cells, which is a tumor. Chemotherapy, radiation, and surgery can help treat cancer. The difference between chemotherapy and radiation is that chemotherapy uses chemicals to destroy the cancer cells. In contrast, radiation uses X-rays or other types of rays to kill them.

Asthma

It is a breathing disorder, which is chronic. This means it lasts for a long time frame. Too much physical pressure, breathing secondhand smoke, or allergies can trigger an attack. Medication and changes in lifestyle can control the asthma.

Diabetes

It occurs when individuals cannot produce enough insulin to use the sugars and starches in food for energy. Insulin is a hormone that is produced in the pancreas to help digest sugar. There is a type 1 and type 2 diabetes. Type 1 diabetes usually occurs with teenagers. Type 2 diabetes usually happens with individuals aged 40 and above. Diabetes can be controlled by having a balanced diet and taking regular medications.

If an individual living with any of these diseases does not take care of themselves or get proper medical treatments then they could die.

Alcohol and the Human Body

Symptoms

1. Headaches

2. Permanent damages to the brain.

3. Hallucinations. Individuals start seeing images that are unreal and their mind is creating the images. This is causing the individual to feel disturbed.

4. Cancer of the esophagus. After eating food, the esophagus is the organ through which food moves.

5. Gastritis ulcers.

6. Cirrhosis of the liver. This is considered a disease in which the healthy cells of the liver begin to die.

7. Extreme tremors found in delirium tremens.

8. Fetal Alcohol Syndrome (FAS), which is characterized by the face and body abnormalities and, in some cases, impaired intellectual facilities.

9. Korsakoff psychosis.

10. Lapse of memory, which are considered "blackouts."

11. Cancer of the mouth.

12. Cancer of the throat.

13. Permanent damage to the central nervous system.

14. Nausea.

15. Inflammation of the pancreas.

16. Combination of alcohol and drugs, such as commonly used sleeping pills, tranquilizers, antibiotics, and aspirin, can be fatal, even when both are taken in non-lethal doses.

Alcohol's Effects on the Body

Alcohol is a depressant. It affects and dismantles the functions of the body and has powerful effects on the entire body. Alcohol is produced by a chemical in some foods. It has no nutrients and just empty calories, which can cause a person to become fat.

What Alcohol Affects?

Alcohol affects the brain by slowing it down and affecting the way a person thinks. As a result, the person usually becomes violent.

Alcohol affects the stomach by damaging the lining and causing open sores.

Alcohol affects the liver, by causing cirrhosis scarring, and destruction of tissue. Cirrhosis can lead to death.

Alcohol affects the blood vessels by widening them and causing the body to lose heat when blood flows to the surface of the body. When this happens then the drinker usually feels warmer than their actual temperature.

The Reactions of People to Alcohol are Influenced by Factors

The Blood Alcohol Level (BAL) is a measure of the amount of alcohol in the bloodstream of the human. The higher the BAL then the more intoxicated the person is considered.

The speed at which an individual drinks alcohol will affect their level of intoxication. It is likely that the symptoms of drinking alcohol will begin faster if the person consumes the alcohol quickly. A symptom can be an individual having headaches.

The amount of alcohol an individual consumes can trigger the speed at which the symptoms will begin.

The weight of an individual can affect how quickly the symptoms of the alcohol will begin within the body.

The amount of food an individual has consumed can react with the alcohol to start certain and negative effects within the body such as regurgitating.

The mood of an individual such as if he or she is happy or sad can work with the alcohol to start the negative effects within the body.

If a consumer has taken other drugs or smoked and later, he or she consumes alcohol then it is likely that the negative effects within the body will begin faster.

Reasons for Drinking Alcohol

Individuals think drinking alcohol will make them feel more grown up or others will view them as being more of an adult.

Individuals may drink due to negative peer pressure from classmates and/or friends and they want to fit in with the crowd.

They may drink thinking such will allow for them to escape their problems in life or overcome their stress and/or depression.

The final common reason why some individuals drink alcohol is because of negative influence from family members. For example, some family members may drink around them and they may develop the impression that it is normal to drink alcohol especially if they are young. Young individuals may not know about all the negative effects of alcohol on the body.

There is no legitimate reason for drinking alcohol.

Reasons to Not Drink Alcohol

Reasons Not to Drink

Drinking is illegal if an individual is under the legal drinking age of their state.

Drinking gets in the way.

Drinking is not fun.

Drinking is not smart.

Drinking does not solve problems.

Drinking disappoints others such as family members and friends.

Drinking makes the user feel guilty.

Drinking harms health.

Ways to Avoid Drinking

Choose a way that speaks the truth for the individual.

Avoid situations in which people are drinking.

Suggest alternatives to drinking such as drinking soda or a type of juice.

True friends support and respect the decisions of their peers, colleagues, and other friends.

Signs of Drug Misuse and Drug Abuse

Drug Misuse: Not taking or using medicines in the way that the doctor has ordered.

-Taking a medicine for longer than prescribed.

-Not taking a medicine for the full time prescribed.

-Changing the amount of a medicine an individual is taking or mixing medicines without asking the doctor or medical professional.

-Using an old prescription medicine without checking with the doctor.

-Using a medicine prescribed for another individual.

Drug Abuse: Using drugs in ways that are unhealthy or illegal.

-Using a medicine for non-medical purposes.

-Swallowing or breathing a substance that was not meant to enter the body.

-Using a drug in a way that is harmful physically, mentally, or socially to the individual.

Understand these Terms

Drug: A substance other than food that changes the structure or function of the body or mind.

Medicine: Drugs that are used to prevent, control, or cure diseases or other conditions.

Over-the-counter (OTC) medicine: Medicines that are considered safe enough to be taken without a written order (prescription) from a doctor.

Prescription medicine: Medicines that can be sold only with a written order from a doctor.

Medicine

A drug is considered any substance that changes the function or structure of the body or mind. They are used to prevent or treat diseases, illnesses, and other conditions.

Prescription medicines cannot be taken or sold with a written order from a physician. This is because it is possible some individuals may abuse or misuse the medicines.

Over-the-counter (OTC) medicines are safe enough to be purchased and taken without an order from the medical physician.

FDA is an abbreviation for the Food and Drug Administration. This is the government agency that tests medicines.

A prescription is a type of medicine for which an individual needs the written order of the doctor.

When an individual uses a medicine for non-medical purposes or uses a medicine after the expiration date then this is usually a sign of drug abuse. Medicines that have expired should always be discarded.

A side effect is a reaction to the medicine other than the reaction that was intended.

Medicines can enter the body through mucous membranes, the skin, or veins.

Inhaled medicine enters the lungs and then moves into the bloodstream.

If a medicine no longer gives an individual the same effect then the individual may have developed tolerance. Tolerance means the body has been used to the effects of the medicine and needs it in a greater quantity for the body to have the same effect.

Preparations of dead or weakened germs that cause the immune system to produce antibodies are called vaccines.

Medicine injected into the muscle immediately enters the bloodstream. This is why doctors sometimes have to give injections.

Three Common Types

- Vaccines are medicines that prevent diseases.

- Asprin and medicines similar to aspirin are used to relieve pain but individuals should be careful when taking them. If individuals are still having pain after taking such medicine then they should not take more before consulting with a doctor.

- Antibiotics are medicines that reduce or kill harmful bacteria in the body.

Stages of Addiction

1. First occasional usage of the drug.

2. Regular usage of the drug.

3. Intensified usage of the drug.

4. The individual develops total dependence on the drug.

Substance Addiction

Types of Addiction

A. Physical dependence: The body needs the substance simply to properly function. Drugs that usually cause an individual to develop physical dependence are stimulants, depressants, narcotics, and alcohol.

B. Psychological dependence: The person believes that they need the drug to feel good. Drugs that usually cause psychological dependence are marijuana and alcohol.

How to Break an Addiction to Alcohol or Drugs

A. Admit the problem.

B. Stop using the drug.

C. Decide to change.

D. Take responsibility for actions.

Stages of Addiction

A. First use.

B. Regular use.

C. Intensified use.

D. Total dependence.
*An individual feels as though they cannot live without the substance.

Support Groups for Substance Abusers

A. Alcoholics Anonymous (AA).

B. Narcotics Anonymous.

Other sources of help: Hospitals, mental health agencies, special counselors, and drug abuse treatment centers.

Help for Families of Substance Abusers

A. Alateen: Helps children of alcoholic parents learn how to cope with problems at home.

B. Al-Anon: Helps husbands, wives, and friends of alcoholics learn more about alcoholism.

C. Nar-Anon: Holds meetings for families of drug addicts.

Golden Rule

Individuals who are trying to break their addiction to any type of drug or tobacco should avoid enablers. Enablers are people who support the individual using the dangerous substance. For example, if the mother of an individual gave them cigars to smoke then the mother would be considered an enabler. The individual should avoid the mother or tell the mother to stop handing them cigars. In addition, individuals should not start using another drug for the purpose of quitting using a current drug. For example, an individual who is trying to stop drinking alcohol should not start smoking cigars. In some cases, using another drug to quit using the current drug will strengthen the overall addiction and cause the individual to greatly use both drugs. The individual is increasing their likelihood of developing some type of horrible condition and passing away faster.

Treatment for Alcoholism

There are 3 stages an individual undergoes as they become an alcoholic. An alcoholic is an addicted user of alcohol and drinks it excessively feeling dependent on it.

Stage #1
A person starts using alcohol to relax or relive stress or pain. For this reason, the drinker begins to make excuses about his or her drinking habits.

Stage #2
The drinker is often absent from their job or school. This is because their body is developing a need to drink increasing amounts of alcohol so they will spend most of their time in doing so.

Stage #3
Drinking becomes an important part of the life of the individual. Without alcohol, the drinker feels mental and physical pain. As a result, their drinking habits are out of control.

1 in 4 families within the United States are affected by alcoholism. Alcoholism is the strong physical and mental need to have alcohol. This unhealthy need can be considered a disease. All users must understand the steps to recover from alcoholism.

#1 Tip for Recovery
The alcoholic must admit to themselves that they have a drinking problem and seek help so they can recover. Alcoholics are unlikely to recover if they are stubborn and ignore the fact they have a problem.

#2 Seek a Support Group
-Al-Anon: Helps family members and friends of alcoholics

-Alateen: Helps young people cope with the fact they have a family member or friend who is an alcoholic.

-Alcoholics Anonymous: An alcoholic would participate in a session with other alcoholics and they would all admit to their problems. Strategies would be discussed to help stop the excessive consumption of alcohol. There would be a counselor at all the sessions to help guide them.

*There may be more support groups in society. An individual could do an internet search to find all the groups or check with a friend, school, or work official. However, an individual should never pay money to join a group because it is likely to be a scam. The groups that were mentioned are free.

Ways an Individual can help an Alcoholic

-Tell the parents of the alcoholic or anonymously inform a school counselor of the problem if the individual consuming alcohol is below 21.
-Not give them alcohol.
-Make them realize alcohol can kill them.
-Provide information about groups that can help them end the drinking problems.
-Make them realize they have much potential to achieve success in life and drinking alcohol will ruin all their chances.
-Make the alcoholic aware they can no longer be friends or see each other if they continue their bad habit.

Reasons not to Drink (Reinforced)

It is illegal if an individual is under the legal drinking age (all states have different ages).
It gets in the way.
It is not fun.
It is not smart or intelligent.
It does not solve problems.
It disappoints others and makes the user feel guilty and wrong.
It harms the health and body.

Alcoholism to Recovery

Alcoholism- Stages to Complete Intoxication

Stage One

The drinker begins to use alcohol to relieve stress and to cope with the pressures of life.

Stage Two

The body of the drinker develops a need for consuming increasing amounts of alcohol. The drinker is often absent from school or work but denies there is a problem.

Stage Three

The body of the drinker is strongly addicted and the drinking is now out of control.

Recovery from Intoxication

Step One

The alcoholic admits to having a problem and asks for help.

Step Two

The alcoholic goes through detoxification and begins to regain physical health.

Step Three

The alcoholic receives counseling on how to live without alcohol.

Tobacco and the Body

1. Gum disease.

2. Tooth decay and tooth loss.

3. Bad breath.

4. Oral cancer.

5. Heart disease.

6. Increased risk of fatal breast cancer.

7. Lung cancer.

8. Loss of appetite.

9. Cancer of the pancreas.
*Pancreas is the organ that creates enzymes to help digest food as it enters the small intestine.

10. Bladder cancer.

11. Mineral content of bone is reduced.

12. Delayed wound healing.

13. Raises blood pressure.

14. Cancer of the kidney.

15. Gullet cancer.

16. Increases stomach acid.

17. Systemic arteriosclerosis
*This is a type of heart disease that involves the hardening of the arteries.

18. Chronic bronchitis.

19. Lip cancer.

How Tobacco Smoke Affects the Body

Tobacco smoke can harm smokers and nonsmokers who inhale secondhand smoke. Secondhand smoke is created when an individual smokes near another individual whom breathes it. For example, if Danny's grandmother smokes cigarettes in the bathroom and Danny goes into the bathroom shortly after she is done smoking then he will likely breathe in the secondhand smoke. The secondhand smoke can damage the health conditions of Danny similar to how the health conditions of smokers are damaged. Smokers and breathers of secondhand smoke can develop a condition called emphysema. It happens when the small air sacs in the lungs are damaged or destroyed. Harmful chemicals in the smoke can also cause lung cancer.

The secondhand smoke is carbon monoxide. It reduces the amount of oxygen within the blood and narrows the blood vessels. This means the body organs receive less oxygen and this can be especially dangerous for pregnant women. If their baby does not receive enough oxygen then it is possible the baby could die within the woman. This case is considered the Sudden Infant Death Syndrome (SIDS). The woman could also potentially experience a miscarriage with the baby or cause them to be born with mental or physical abnormalities. These abnormalities are scary.

Nicotine is a chemical within the tobacco that usually causes the addiction to smoking. It travels to the brain and speeds up the functions of the body. This puts more pressure on the heart and can lead to a heart attack.

Tobacco can lead to an individual developing a stomach ulcer. This may cause the stomach to feel sore. Smokers have a greater chance of developing bladder, colon, mouth, and throat cancer.

Smoking may cause the fingers to become stained and yellow. It may cause smokers to get wrinkles earlier than nonsmokers and it stains their teeth. This will look ugly.

The mentioned health problems can be caused by snuff. Snuff is ground tobacco held in the mouth. As a personal analysis, ground tobacco must be very harmful if it is only supposed to be held in the mouth. It raises the question what would happen if an individual swallowed the tobacco. It is likely that the individual will increase their chances of developing bad health conditions. Ideally, if a substance is so powerful it should not be swallowed then an individual should not have it at all and avoid this risk.

Individuals who stop using a drug or tobacco may face painful physical and mental symptoms due. This is because they were dependent on the substance. This stage is called withdrawal. If needed, individuals should get medical help to overcome the withdrawal stage. This is because not being able to withstand the symptoms of the stage may cause them to take the dangerous substance again.

Interesting Facts and Myths about Tobacco

Facts
1. A single puff of cigarette smoke exposes the body to many deadly chemicals.
2. Every year, an increasing number of people are quitting their smoking habit.
3. Smokeless tobacco has harmful effects on the digestive system as well as on the heart and lungs.
4. Smoking can be an expensive habit.
5. There are laws limiting where people may smoke.
6. Smoking weakens the senses of taste and smell of the smoker.
7. Smoking a cigarette is like breathing the exhaust fumes of a car.

Myths
1. Smoking helps people concentrate on their work.
Truth: All the chemicals in tobacco and the secondhand smoke it produces can cause many damaging effects to the body as proven by research. There is no research suggesting that smoking can help individuals achieve better levels of concentration or focus on tasks. If anything, smoking weakens concentration because individuals may start to feel ill when their blood pressure increases, they feel tired, or they cannot properly breathe.

2. Smokers harm only themselves. Therefore, nonsmokers do not need to be concerned.
Truth: When individuals smoke then they do hurt their family members or friends in some aspect. Nonsmokers should be concerned because if they breathe in the secondhand smoke then they could develop serious health conditions such as emphysema or lung cancer. Nonsmokers who are friends with young smokers whom live with their parents should tell their parents about the bad habits. Finally, smokers sometimes become violent towards individuals. For this reason, individuals around smokers should be cautious.

3. Chewing tobacco is not addictive.
Truth: Like the tobacco found in cigars and cigarettes, chewing tobacco has the substance called nicotine. Nicotine causes the individual to develop an addiction to tobacco and feel dependent on it. In fact, it is likely the cigar and cigarette companies know the strong addictive aspect of nicotine. For this reason, they will put nicotine in all or most their products. They want individuals to get addicted to the tobacco so they continue purchasing it and the companies continue making high levels of profit (money).

4. Smoking is an easy habit to break.
Truth: If smoking was an easy habit to break then it should raise the question as to why there are many smoking support groups for smokers to get help. It is not an easy habit to break. To further support this point, the Centers for Disease Control and Prevention

reports smoking causes about 1 of every 5 deaths in the United States every year. It is unlikely 443,000 deaths in the United States would occur if an individual stopping to smoke was an easy habit to break.

5. When a person stops smoking, the body cannot recover.
Truth: Smoking has caused some damage to the body of the smoker for the time they were smoking. However, the bad effects of smoking can partially recover if the person permanently stops smoking, avoids all drugs, exercises, and eats a healthy diet. It is likely the blood pressure of the individual will become normal. This will reduce their chances of having a heart attack. The wrinkles of the individual may start to go away and their teeth will become cleaner of the stains. The breathing functions of the individual will become normal. The recovery is not instant but it will gradually happen as long as an individual remains motivated to stop smoking cigars or cigarettes.

6. A teenager who smokes looks more mature.
Truth: There is no "mature" aspect about smoking especially if an individual is a teenager. If anything, smoking is immature because it shows the teenager is ignorant and they are not aware of all the harmful effects of this bad habit. The teenager is ignorantly ruining their future by smoking. This is because it may cause for them to do poorly in school and get involved with dangerous activities and groups such as gangs. The teenager may become so ill to the point that it is unlikely they will be able to play sports or pursue a career.

7. Filtered cigarettes reduce the amount of tar and nicotine released.
Truth: There is no research suggesting this claim about filtered cigarettes is true. The cigar and cigarette companies know if they do not include the nicotine and tar chemicals within the cigars and cigarettes then they may not be able to make as much profit as possible. This is because it is likely that less people will smoke cigars and cigarettes. Nicotine is the substance that causes the addiction. In addition with the other substances, tar is the substance that causes the relaxing feeling smokers receive while smoking and wanting to receive the same feeling makes them want to smoke again.

8. Smoking for just a few years cannot hurt an individual.
Truth: When an individual smokes, the negative effects of smoking begin happening within the body immediately. The blood pressure begins to increase, blood starts to become unhealthy due to a lack of proper oxygen, the air sacs within the lung start to become damaged, and these effects are minor compared to all the negative effects. The individual could have a heart attack or could permanently damage their lungs at any time. As months pass, the lungs of smokers become increasingly black and ugly. The smoker may struggle to become healthy again if the smoker decides to stop their bad habit.

Abused Drugs

The use of illegal drugs and the abuse of legal medicines can have harmful effects on the physical and mental well-being of the individual.

Stimulants are drugs that speed up the functions of the body and mind. Cocaine is a stimulant and it can cause an individual not to be sleepy, loss of appetite, and be nervous. If an individual injects themselves with cocaine and uses dirty or borrowed needles then they run the risk of becoming infected with HIV or possibly another disease.

Depressants are drugs that slow down the functions of the body and mind.

Narcotics are a group of drugs used to relieve pain.

Anabolic steroids are based on the male hormone called testosterone.

Marijuana is an illegal drug made from the hemp plant. The drug can increase the heart rate and cause panic attacks.

Inhalants are substances whose fumes are breathed in to give the effect of a hallucinogen.

Hallucinogens cause the brain of the user to distort real images. This can cause the user to see and hear objects that are not real but fake.

Drug Classifications

Classification
Stimulants

Drugs
Amphetamine
Cocaine (powder form)
Crack

Effects
-Increases awareness, blood pressure, and heart rate.
-Makes an individual less tired and less hungry.
-It can cause an individual to see delusions.
-The individual may hallucinate.
-Excessively using a stimulant can lead to death.

Classification
Depressants

Drugs
Alcohol
Tranquilizers
*A tranquilizer may be given to an individual who has been raped to help calm them.
Barbiturates

Effects
-Reduces the activity level of the central nervous system.
-Low doses reduce anxiety (nervousness) and/or tension.
-High doses can lead to death.

Classification
Narcotics

Drugs
Codeine
Morphine
Heroin
*Made from Morphine
Opium
Methadone

Effects
-Decrease the pain level of an individual.
-Highly addictive.

Classification
Hallucinogens

Drugs
LSD
PCP (Phencyclidine)
Mescaline
Psilocybin
Marijuana
Hashish

Effects
-It changes the way an individual can see and hear.
-It may cause an individual to get terrified because the sights and sounds are perceived in frightening ways.
-Drugs produce anxiety, panic attacks, psychotic effects, flashbacks, and hallucinations.
-Brain damage can occur with the individual.
-It can lead to death.

Classification
Inhalants

Drugs
Paint thinner
Model glue
Gasoline
Correction fluid
Freon
Aerosol spray

Effects
-It can cause headaches, nausea, and hallucinations.
-An individual may have memory losses, they may get confused, and/or they may become violent.
-Lowers the performance levels of the cardiovascular (heart) and respiratory (breathing) systems.
-Can cause damage to the kidneys, liver, bone marrow, and brain.

Street Drugs

All street drugs are dangerous and illegal in some states.

Marijuana
It changes the mind of the individual to make them feel more relaxed. For this reason, the marijuana has several different chemicals including THC (tetrahydrocannabinol). A more powerful drug derived from the same plant is hashish.

Hallucinogens
Drugs that distort the moods, thoughts, and senses of an individual. Examples of hallucinogens include PCP, LSD, mescaline, and mushrooms.

Designer Drugs
Drugs that are made from chemicals that resemble illegal substances. Ecstasy or MDMA are designer drugs.

Inhalants
Substances whose fumes are sniffed and inhaled to give a soothing effect to the individual. Examples of inhalants are glue, spray paint, gasoline, nitrites, nitrous oxide, and the scent from some markers.

Marijuana

Smoking marijuana causes breathing problems. As support, users of marijuana have more colds and upper respiratory system problems.

Marijuana negatively affects the brain and body.
-Short-term memory losses.
-Loss of the ability to concentrate.
-Slows coordination and reflexes.
-Affects the ability to judge distance, speed, and reaction time- these abilities are important in playing sports or even riding a bike.

There is more tar is marijuana smoke than in tobacco smoke. This may cause the lungs to become more black, ugly, and unhealthy.

Marijuana users have an increased risk of developing cancer.

Marijuana smoke contains 50% to 70% more of some cancer causing chemicals than tobacco smoke.

Drugs that are Misused and Abused

Narcotics

Specific drugs that are obtainable only by prescription and are used to relieve some type of pain.

Examples of narcotics include morphine, heroin, and codeine.

Stimulants

Drugs that speed up the functions of the body.

Examples of stimulants include cocaine, crack cocaine, amphetamines, and caffeine.

Depressants

Drugs that slow down the functions and reactions of the body.

Examples of depressants include tranquilizers, hypnotics, and barbiturates.

Drugs and Alcohol Review

1. Using a medicine incorrectly is drug misuse. An example of drug misuse is when an individual does not follow the label directions on the medicine bottle and takes a higher amount of medicine than what is needed.

2. Drugs that relieve an individual of pain are morphine, heroin, and codeine. These drugs fall into the category of narcotics.

3. Alcohol slows down the thinking and movements of an individual because it is a depressant.

4. People will react differently when they drink alcohol depending upon how much food they have eaten and possibly other drugs and/or beverages they have consumed.

5. A person who has been drinking alcohol can feel warmer than their actual body temperature.

6. Alcohol can cause cirrhosis, which is the destruction of the liver cells.

7. Drugs that speed up the functions of the body such as cocaine and amphetamines are stimulants.

8. Expecting mothers can prevent their babies from being born with fetal alcohol syndrome by not drinking alcohol.

9. Drugs that slow down the functions of the body such as tranquilizers and barbiturates are depressants.

10. Substances besides food that change the function of the mind or body are drugs.

11. The mental or physical need for a drug, tobacco, or other substance is addiction.

Factors that Compose the Environment

Living Things (Biotic Factors)
1. Plants
2. Animals
3. Other people

Nonliving Things (Abiotic Factors)
1. Air
2. Water
3. Soil

Safety

To act in a safe manner, an individual must avoid taking unnecessary risks. Risks are chances a person takes that could be harmful. An example of a risky situation is an individual riding a motorcycle without a helmet.

There are three guidelines that will help an individual avoid risks and act safely.

1. Individuals should not give into negative peer pressure.

2. Individuals should think before they act.

3. Individuals should know their own limits.

These guidelines will help the individual break the accident chain. The accident chain has five parts.

1. The situation or problem.

2. The unsafe habit.

3. The unsafe act or action.

4. The accident.

5. The results of the accident.

A hazard is a possible source of harm. Two examples of hazards are electrical cutlets and cluttered stairways. Individuals should avoid hazards to best protect their lives.

Violence

People who use drugs, tobacco, and/or alcohol can become violent and not be able to control all their actions.

In a tense situation, if people cannot control their anger then it can lead to violence.

Violence is the use of physical or mental force to inflict harm on an individual.

Causes of violence can include anger, usage of drugs, peer pressure, prejudice, and possession of a weapon such as a gun.

Prejudice can lead to violent acts called hate crimes. Prejudice is a judgment or opinion about someone that is not based on facts, information, or knowledge of the person.

The pressure that teens put on each other to be part of a group is called peer pressure. In some cases, these groups are considered to be gangs.

Some teens think using guns will impress peers and make them feel powerful and impress other peers.

In some gangs, they use guns to perform drive-by shootings. This is when an individual shoots another individual while driving a car. The purpose of drive-by shootings is to cause harm to an individual.

Some gangs participate in carjacking. This is when a person steals an automobile by threatening the driver with a weapon.

Outdoor Safety

To be safe outdoors, it is important to plan ahead and know the outdoor safety rules. For this purpose, it is recommended individuals use the buddy system. The buddy system is an agreement between two or more people to stay together and watch as well as care for the safety of each other. In the case of an emergency or problem, the individual and their buddy can help and support each other.

In the Water

The most important task an individual can do to be safe is to learn how to properly swim.

In an individual thinks they are drowning then they should use the technique called the drowning prevention to save themselves.

If an individual is in cold water for too long then they can develop hypothermia. This is when the temperature of the body significantly drops.

Hiking and Camping

To be safe while hiking and camping, individuals should take the proper equipment with them.

They should never camp alone and wear appropriate clothing to protect themselves against insects and bruises.

Individuals should stay in specified campsites and/or areas so they can avoid dangerous plants, snakes, or insects. They should not cook in the tents.

At the end of the trip, they should put out all the campfires.

Winter Sports

The best way for an individual to protect themselves from the cold is to wear the proper clothing.

In extreme cold, the skin of an individual can freeze and this can cause frostbite. Frostbite is an injury damage underneath the skin.

Bicycle Safety

Individuals should practice defensive driving and this means obeying traffic rules and watching out for other road users.

Make sure the bike has the proper safety gear.

Ride on the right side of the road.

Use lights and reflective clothing when riding after dark. If possible, ride with another individual during and after the dark. This is called using the buddy system.

Avoid loose clothing that could get caught in the chain.

Always wear a helmet.

Weather Emergencies

Floods are the most common natural disasters. Some floods take days to develop and others develop within minutes.

Safety Tips with Floods

Individuals should listen to the local radio and/or television stations for the news. They should not walk or ride in a vehicle through water.

Earthquakes

An earthquake is the result of the grounds shaking as their rocks are moving below the surface.

Safety Tips with Earthquakes

If an individual is inside in an earthquake then they should go inside their house or shelter. If an individual is outside in an earthquake then they should stand out in the open.

Hurricanes and Tornadoes

A hurricane is a strong windstorm with driving rain.

A tornado is a whirling, funnel-shaped thunderstorm that drops from the sky to the ground.

Safety Tips with Hurricanes and Tornadoes

In a hurricane or tornado, individuals who live on the coast should go to an island for maximum safety if such is possible. If an individual is outdoors during a tornado or hurricane then they should lie flat in a ditch and cover themselves with a protective item such as a blanket or some type of clothing.

First Aid in Five Minutes

First aid is care given to an injured or ill individual in an emergency or accident until regular medical care can be supplied.

Follow theses steps in the first five minutes immediately if an individual needs first aid. These steps could really make a difference in saving their life.

1. Rescue the victim through any means possible. Move the victim only if they are in an unsafe area or location.

2. The individual should check the breathing activity of the victim. If their airway is blocked then the individual should try and clear it. Individuals should not worry about getting germs. Turn the head of the victim to the side to prevent choking on whatever it is that is blocking their airway.

3. Control the bleeding of the victim. If the victim is losing a large amount of blood then the individual should apply direct pressure.

4. Get medical help immediately. In many cases, an individual can dial 911 or have another individual with a cell phone dial it for the purpose of reaching the Emergency Medical Services department.

First Aid for Burns

First-degree Burn
A burn in which only the outer layer of the skin is affected.

Treatment
1. Submerge the burned area in cold water.
2. Warm and wrap the burned area loosely in a clean, dry dressing.

Second-degree Burn
A serious burn that damages the first and second layers of skin.

Treatment
1. Submerge the burned area in cold water.
2. Wrap the burn loosely in a clean and dry dressing.
3. Evaluate the burned area.

Third-degree Burn
A very serious burn that destroys skin and may affect fat, nerves, tissues, and bones.

Treatment
1. Call for medical help.
2. Cover the burned area with a clean dressing.
3. Elevate the feet and arms.
4. Give small amounts of fluids.

First Aid for Choking

Self

Gives the signs of choking.

Perform abdominal thrusts, which are quick, upward pulls into the diaphragm to force out the substances blocking the airway.

Adults and Other Children

Ask "are you choking?"

Perform abdominal thrusts.

Infants and Young Children

Give the victim several blows with the heel of the hand between the shoulder blades.

Perform chest thrusts, which are quick pressures into the middle of the breastbone belonging to the individual.

Repeat the techniques as necessary for any case.

Rescue Breathing Steps

Rescue breathing is when an individual substitutes for the normal breathing of a victim. They force air into the lungs of the victim. They are trying to free the victim of whatever is blocking their airways.

1. Look, listen, and feel to see if the victim is breathing on their own.

2. Open the airway of the victim.

3. Pinch the nostrils of the victim shut.

4. The individual should place their mouth over the mouth of the victim.

5. Give two full breaths.

6. Pause to let the air flow out.

7. Repeat.

Steps to Treat a Choking Victim

Choking is a condition that occurs when the airway of an individual is blocked.

1. Ask "Are you choking?"

2. Stand behind the victim.

3. The individual should wrap the arms around the waist of the victim.

4. The individual should put their fist against the abdomen of the victim. The individual should put their fist with the other hand.

5. Give quick upward thrusts.

6. Repeat.

Safety Review

Potentially harmful chances a person could take, like riding a bike, are called risks. The use of force to harm someone is called violence.

Individuals can avoid being a victim of crime by walking with confidence and purpose. It is very important to use the buddy system when outdoors. An individual is to stay together and watch for the safety of each other. If there is an emergency, an individual can help each other.

Risks and Prevention

The most important task an individual can do to be safe in the water is to learn how to swim.

Frostbite is the freezing of the skin.

A tornado warning is issued when a tornado is in the area.

If an individual is inside a building during an earthquake, they should not go outside.

If an individual swallows some type of substance or food they think is poisonous or witnesses another individual doing so, they should immediately contact a Poison Control Center.

When buying products, it is best to look for ones that have the recycling symbol.

Helping the Environment

In order for individuals to be healthy, they must live in a healthy world. All individuals should work together to achieve this goal and here are some strategies to follow as much as possible in everyday life. They all benefit the planet Earth.

1. Rather than riding in an automobile, walk or ride a bike.

2. Turn off radios, lights, and television sets when they are not being used.

3. Turn down the heat when no individual is at the house or building location. Doing so also saves money.

4. Do not run the dishwasher or washing machine unless there is a full load of clothes.

5. Do not waste the water by leaving it running or by taking unnecessarily long showers.

6. Discard trash properly rather than liter the surroundings.

7. Keep radio and television sets turned low rather than pollute the environment by having them on too loud.

8. Recycle paper, plastic, aluminum, and glass.

9. Volunteer time to make the environment cleaner and safer.

10. Put litter in its place.

11. Choose products in reusable or recyclable packages.

12. Use public transportation when possible.

13. Use non-aerosol sprays.

14. Use non-disposable materials instead of paper plates and cups.

15. Avoid smoking.

Air Pollution

Air Pollution

-Burning fossil fuels, such as oil, coal, and natural gas.

-Fires.

-Chemicals such as pesticides and chlorofluorocarbons.

-Health chemicals such as shortness of breath, sneezing, itchy eyes, asthma, and emphysema.

-Ozone destruction. Ozone is a form of oxygen.

-Acid rain: Rain or snow that is more acidic than normal.

-Smog: Yellow-brown haze that forms when sunlight reacts with impurities in car exhaust.

-Greenhouse effect: Trapping of heat by carbon dioxide and other gases in the air.

Conservation

- It is very important to conserve (save) nonrenewable resources. These are substances that cannot be replaced once they are used by a consumer.

- Conservation is the saving of resources.

- Resources can be conserved through recycling, which is changing items in some aspect and using them again for some purpose.

- Resources can be conserved through precycling, which is reducing wastes before it occurs.

Solid Waste Disposal

Solid Waste

Amount created each year is about 2 million tons.

Disposal Options

Landfills, which are places where wastes are dumped and buried.

Disadvantages

-Only certain wastes can be dumped in them.
-They are unpleasant and unsightly.
-They take up space.

Burning, this is done in special furnaces called incinerators.

Disadvantages

-They are expensive to build and operate.
-Only certain wastes can be burned safely.
-Smoke and ashes may harm the environment.

Works Cited

*Most of the facts presented throughout the book were collected from the Centers for Disease Control and Prevention and *Teen Health* unless otherwise indicated on the chapter.

ALAW Air Quality Monitoring Survey; 2006.

Behavioral Risk Factor Surveillance System, Washington State Department of Health; 2005 and 2006.

"Can Stress Affect Your Health Triangle?" *Healthy Living*. Web. 25 July 2013.

Centers for Disease Control and Prevention (CDC), Office on Smoking and Health. Best practices for comprehensive tobacco control programs—2007. Atlanta: CDC; 2007.

Centers for Disease Control and Prevention (CDC), National Center for Chronic Disease Prevention and Health Promotion, Office on Smoking and Health. Reducing tobacco use: A report of the Surgeon General. Atlanta: CDC; 2000.

"Improving Emotional Health." *Strategies and Tips for Good Mental Health*.

Web. 25 July 2013.

Works Cited (Continued)

Merki, Mary Bronson., Michael J. Cleary, Betty M. Hubbard, and Dinah Zike.

    Teen Health. New York, NY: Glencoe/McGraw-Hill, 2005. Print.

"Risk Factors to Health." *(AIHW)*. Web. 25 June 2013.

"The Habits of Healthy People." *Nutrition*. Web. 25 June 2013.

Acknowledgements

I never thought in my life I would write a third book but I was given the encouragement to do so by several people who mean the world to me. Although there are many names, it does not mean I typed up a random list. Any success with this book would not have been possible without the support of these people who are the most brilliant and amazing individuals anyone can meet. I mean this from my heart.

University High School International Baccalaureate Class of 2011

Kathleen Acevedo
Joshua Aguilar
Marissa Alonso
Chynna Bambico
Christine Barbosa
Iman Boudlal
Maria Carrasco
Matthew Castner
Ian Chin-See
Caisey Cole
Sean Conte
Alan Dang
Kim Dang
Ashley de Haas
Glisairis Depena
Melissa Dinh
Elizabeth Eby
Melissa Eby
Manu Elias
Elizabeth Escobedo
Rosana Eustache
Cristina Flores
Victoria Flores
Reimar Francisco
Natalia Frias
Carla Gabaldon-Torrents
Ashley Garrett
Lemuel Gorion
Matthew Gorion
Lizbeth Guzman
Richard Haddock
Alinnette Hernandez
Brittany Jean-Pierre
Paul Jenny

Peter Jiang
Parth Kataria
Elizabeth Kilian
Elizabeth Knorr
Brandon Laines
Vladimir Llarch
Daniel Lockaby
Timothy McCarthy
Rachel McLeod
Tanisa McLeod
Tanisa McMillian
Christopher McNamara
Jillian Mendoza
Rebecca Miller
Deandra Modeste
Cameron Neilson
Nicole Neilson
Jennifer Newton
Paul Nguyen
Pete Oshkolup
Samuel Pan
Mitchell Quach
Erika Ramirez
Suraj Ramnarain
Kirstin Raymond
Paola Rodriguez
Jared Ruddell
Angel Santiago
Friedrich Schulte
Stephanie Silvius
Charlotte Smith
Kenlyn Soucy
Matthew Stover
Roberto Telleria
Daniel Toro
Francine Vassell
Jabril Vilmenay
Nadia Williams
Michelle Windish
Alexis Wood
Sheran Xavier
Ashish Yamdagni

I want to acknowledge two special people. During their lives, they made positive impacts to the lives of many including myself and they are Kelly McConnell, who was an inspiring student, at University High School, part of the International Baccalaureate class of 2009, and Rebecca DeJeasus, who was an administrator and loved teacher at University High School.

2012-2013 The Art and Phyllis Grindle Honors Institute at Seminole State College of Florida

Adriana Tartaglia
Alexandra Worthen
Ali Hussein Yusufali
Alyxis White
Amanda Leigh Mullens
Ana Zuccarini
Anayjay Sparrow
Andre Vega
Andrew Wexler
Angela Dowe-Warren
Ashley Thompson
Austin Gilbert
Austin Kent
Austin Mittan
Austin Wheeler
Brandon Hart
Brian Qualls
Bridget Henry
Bryan Malave
Callme Sally
Cameron Krane
Charles Bilyue
Chelsea Ann Carrera
Chelsea Honeycutt
Christen Fraas
Christopher Posey
Colin Jaye
Crystal Lamson
Daniel Fitzsimons
Devin Walker
Diane Castillo
Dominic Homac
Elisa Carvalho
Elise Pearson
Estefania Trujillo
Fatema Hassanali
Fiorella Gallo
Grace Love
Heather Fox
Jacqueline Stough
James Herzig

Jessica Flachner
Jessica Viera
Joshua Debaere
Joshua Nawrocki
Katie Odell
Ken DeMoya
Kevin Anderson
Khadija Tufail
Kiersten Connor
Kristina Dingeman
Luis Martinez
Maggie Wolff
Matthew Quinones
Medge Parcily
Mell Leonard
Michael McCloskey
Miguel Carvajal
Nicole Brown-Goldman
Nikolas Schulz
Devi Persaud
Phillip Martin
Pooja Salooja
Ratna Okhai
Richard Christel
Ricky Ashby
Sarina Lambert
Sean Moskal
Sergio Almarez
Shacquilla Thompson
Simone Bodecker
Tarik Hamiliton
Tucker Crawford
Vanessa Karpf

My Recognition of Excellence

   Throughout my academic career, I have had the honor of being educated by some of the best teachers in the world. They have helped nurture my advanced academic skills and thinking, which I have reflected throughout my book.

Riverdale Elementary School in Orlando, Florida
(Class of 2004 Graduate)

Principal
Ms. Sylvia Lorraine Boyd

Teachers
Albert Cervellera
Amy Keenan Pruett
Cheryl Smith
Connie Robbins
Debbie Arthur
Donna Cosio
Jack T. Warren
Keaton Schreiner
Lea Anne Moore
Margaret Ragley
Naomi Montilla
Patty McKenna
Sharon Komperda
Susan Curtis
Terri Davidson
Timothy Brewer
Vonda Daniels
Wendy Clyde

Odyssey Middle School in Orlando, Florida
(Class of 2007 Graduate)

Principals
Dr. Christopher Bernier

Mrs. Patricia Bowen-Painter

Teachers
Another Dunem
Becky Jones
Dana Hopper
David Santiago
Dominic Eckhoff
Holly Hodges
Jennifer McConkey
Jiae Dy
Josh Counce
Karen D.Angelo
Kimberly Jenkins
Kimela Graves
Laura Richardson
Linda Torres
Lisa McChesney
Michael Cush
Michael Rochkind
Maxima Harmon
Richard Gotham
Sandra Fleming
Scott Evans
Steve Wise
Suzanne Hakimipour
Timothy Douglas
Windy Lopez

A very special thanks to my science teacher, Dana Hopper, I met Mrs. Hopper the day I first began my journey at Odyssey. She is one of the most motivating teachers a student could ever meet. Through her humor, it is so easy for her to make any student love class. I joined her Science Olympiad club and then followed her when she started a new club with Mr. Dunem called "Science Technology Club."

University High School in Orlando, Florida
(International Baccalaureate class of 2011 Graduate)

Principal
Dr. Michael Armbruster

Teachers
Chris Burley
Dora Paz
Doug Klinkerman
Earl Rowland
Eric Saxon
Frank Valenza
John Bruehl
Kathleen Richardville
Lee Ann Spillane
Lisa Tempest
Martha Heine
Melissa Juergens
Mimi Mendez
Oswald Thomas
Philip Rohleder
Ross Klongerbo
Sejal Jagirdar
Sherry Viersen
Stephen Richardville
Teresa Middleton
Timothy Arnold

A very special thanks to my Latin teacher, Philip Rohleder, I met Mr. Rohleder the day I began at University High. I had his Latin course for all four wonderful years and although I struggled, Mr. Rohleder continued pushing me academically and I was able to learn many new skills perfecting my language skills. He is the only teacher I have had for four wonderful years of my life and I cannot thank him enough for being there for his students.

Seminole State College of Florida in Oviedo, Florida
(The Art & Phyllis Grindle Honors Institute class of 2012 Graduate)

President
Dr. E. Ann McGee

Vice President
Dr. Marcia Roman

Dean of the Arts and Sciences
Dr. Laura Ross

Guidance Counselor
Rebecca Lorenzana

Professors
Alan Kraft
Baboucar Jobe
Chris Wright
Collin Morgan
Debra Socci
Diane Wenzel
George Bernard
Howard Sonn
Jeffrey Smith
Jeri Rogers
Kevin Konecny
Laura Dickinson
Mary Dettman
Melissa Bork
Monique Byrnes
Rachel Braaten
Sarah Hernandez
Susan Bell
Teresa Walsh

2012 – 2013 Phi Beta Lambda Chapter at Seminole State College of Florida

During my college adventures, I have been blessed to befriend some of the most brilliant individuals in the world. These individuals have the intellect and motivation to make many contributions to the world and I consider them all to be my future business partners. We hope to combine our minds to start some major type of organization or business. Together, we proudly form the 2012 – 2013 Phi Beta Lambda chapter at the Oviedo campus of Seminole State College of Florida!

Alexandra Buitron
Ashley Jennings
Ashley Jones
Chris Fidrick
Devin Walker
Kelcie Rebecca Rivera
Lena Colon
Levi Chambers
Mercedes Tamayo
Miguel Rodriguez
Vincent Danisi

Friends of Recognition

One fear I think any new college student faces is whether or not people will accept them and they will not be a social outcast. I had this same fear when I came to Seminole State College after graduating from University High School because I knew no one at the school. I was blessed to befriend these amazing people and they are friends who come only once in a lifetime but last forever. I believe one of the keys behind success is for an individual to associate themselves with other successful individuals. For this reason, I am so proud to consider all these people to be my future business partners and lifetime colleagues. Thank you so much.

Ali Hussein Yusufali
Christopher Posey
Jacky Menelas
Ken DeMoya
Lucdwin Luck
Ricky Ashby
Smit Vadvala
Stannon McCreary
Steven Johnson
Tony Rojas

Dedication to Dr. Debra J. Socci

I want to express a heart-warmed thank you to my favorite professor, Honors director, and role model, Dr. Debra Socci, for encouraging me to write this book and make the best decision in my life by joining the Honors program. I still remember the first day I called her asking about joining Honors and she asked me to come into her office, take a writing test about sayings from motivational speakers, and I was so nervous. When I graduated University High School, I was unsure of my career path but thanks to Dr. Socci, I was able to fully unlock my passion for Finance and Business. She helped organize my financial seminars, informed the Seminole State media department who then did a story on me that got picked up by the Fox 35 news station, and granted me the opportunity to do one of the seminars at the Florida Collegiate Honors Conference.

I was able to win several Honors scholarships thanks to her recommendations. I have made connections with several amazing professors that along with her have helped me grow as both a student and person. For this reason, my negative perception of community colleges had changed and now I am an advocate that attending a community college is the best financial decision that can be made by a student. Dr. Socci taught Biology at the University of South Florida, conducted award-winning brain pathology research, and earned a Ph.D. She has been at Seminole State College since 2001 and with so much professional experience and a passion for learning like no other; Dr. Socci brings a strong foundation to the Art & Phyllis Grindle Honors Institute.

There are so many positive words that can be used to describe Dr. Debra Socci. Whenever a student or professor needs her or has a problem then she is there for them. It is so admirable how dedicated she is in helping students achieve their dreams. She has prepared me so well to take on bigger challenges in life. Even after graduating Seminole State, I hope to keep in contact with Dr. Socci so I can continue following her guidance and mature into a leader only the Art & Phyllis Grindle Honors Institute can bring to the world.